100 Low-Carb Recipes for the Foods You Crave—Minus the Ingredients You Don't!

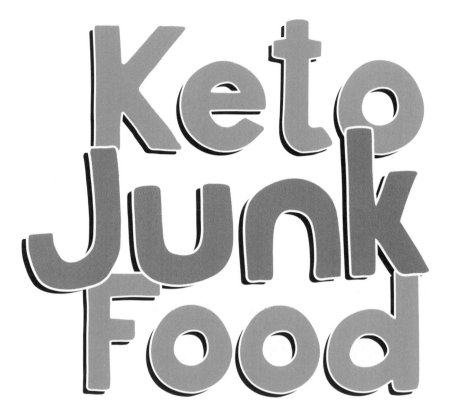

Keto Junk Food

FAITH GORSKY AND LARA CLEVENGER, MSH, RDN, CPT

ADAMS MEDIA

New York • London • Toronto • Sydney • New Delhi

Aadamsmedia

Adams Media
An Imprint of Simon & Schuster, Inc.
100 Technology Center Drive
Stoughton, Massachusetts 02072

First Adams Media trade paperback edition November 2021

ADAMS MEDIA and colophon are trademarks of Simon & Schuster.

For information about special discounts for bulk purchases, please contact Simon & Schuster Special Sales at 1-866-506-1949 or business@simonandschuster.com.

The Simon & Schuster Speakers Bureau can bring authors to your live event. For more information or to book an event contact the Simon & Schuster Speakers Bureau at 1-866-248-3049 or visit our website at www.simonspeakers.com.

Interior design by Priscilla Yuen
Photographs by James Stefiuk

Manufactured in the United States of America

2 2022

Library of Congress Cataloging-in-Publication Data
Names: Gorsky, Faith, author. | Clevenger, Lara, author.
Title: Keto junk food / Faith Gorsky and Lara Clevenger, MSH, RDN, CPT.
Description: First Adams Media trade paperback edition. | Stoughton, MA: Adams Media, 2021. | Includes index.
Identifiers: LCCN 2021032182 | ISBN 9781507216521 (pb) | ISBN 9781507216538 (ebook)
Subjects: LCSH: Ketogenic diet. | Low-carbohydrate diet. | Junk food.
Classification: LCC RC374.K46 G67 2021 | DDC 613.2/833--dc23
LC record available at https://lccn.loc.gov/2021032182

ISBN 978-1-5072-1652-1
ISBN 978-1-5072-1653-8 (ebook)

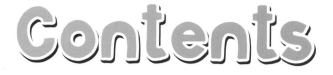

Contents

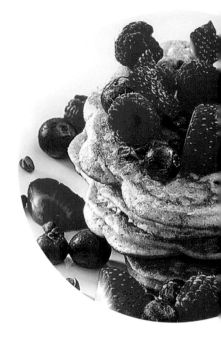

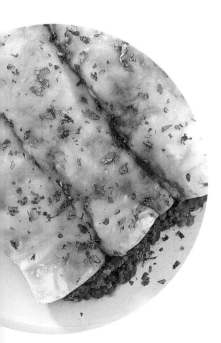

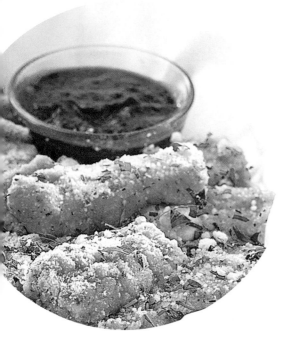

CHAPTER 6
Taqueria Night 99

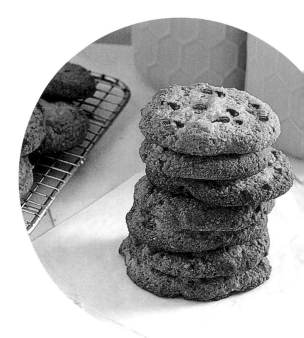

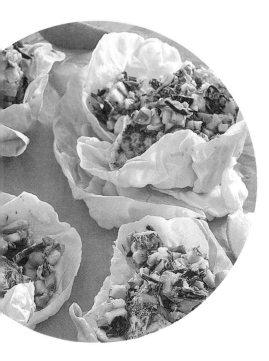

CHAPTER 7
Bakery Favorites 117

CHAPTER 8

Ice Cream Shop 137

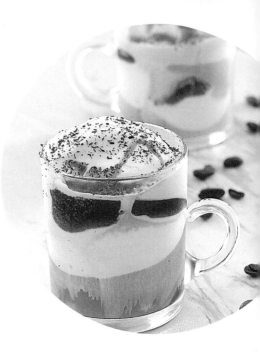

CHAPTER 9

Happy Hour Drinks & Bar Bites 153

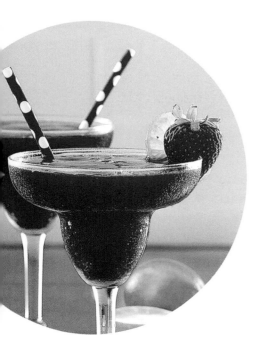

Introduction

*Salty, crunchy snacks; sweet candy, cookies, and ice cream;
greasy fried foods and burgers!*

There's something incredibly satisfying about eating high-carb foods like this, which is why they're called junk foods, right? Now that you're keto, you probably thought you had to give up these foods for good. Well, think again!

Keto Junk Food will bring those delicious and decadent snacks and treats back into your life so you can not only satisfy your junk food cravings but also feed your loved ones nourishing snacks and meals! It's yet more proof that eating keto doesn't have to be restrictive and you don't have to feel deprived.

Inside, you'll find one hundred keto-approved junk food recipes that can easily and mindfully fit into your ketogenic lifestyle. Our decadent recipes, such as Classic Cheesecake, Edible Cookie Dough, Texas Chocolate Sheet Cake, and Cookies and Cream Milkshakes, don't have to be indulgences. Foods like Garlic Breadsticks, Chocolate Chip Pancakes, "Mac" and Cheese Bites, Keto Lo Mein, and Club Sandwich Roll-Ups don't have to break the carb bank. Pizza night (hello, Triple Cheese Pizza, Onion Rings, Buffalo Wings, and Mozzarella Sticks) can still happen. Asian takeout can still be a family favorite, with updated recipes for Sesame Chicken, Singapore Noodles, and Keto Pad Thai. Even Taco Tuesdays are still on the table with our Chips and Queso, Carnitas Tacos, 7-Layer Dip, and Chicken Fajitas. And you should always save room for a keto dessert, especially when Brownie Bites, Strawberry Shortcake Cake Roll, a Tiramisu Parfait, or a Kitchen Sink Ice Cream Sundae is involved.

And this cookbook makes meal prep easy, too, with recipes that freeze well (like Savory Waffles), dishes that are easy to repurpose (such as Ground Beef Taco Meat), and dishes that reheat like a dream (get on those Club Sandwich Roll-Ups and Chicken Tikka Masala).

These keto junk food recipes will easily fit into your lifestyle while still keeping your macros on target with minimal effort. Get ready to fall in love with junk food all over again!

CHAPTER 1

Introduction to Junk Food on the Keto Diet

Switching to a keto diet can be a challenge, especially when you're used to eating sweets and treats and maybe even junk food frequently. Fortunately, the recipes in this book will provide you with low-carb, great-tasting recipes to swap out with your old sugary ones so that you can seamlessly transition into a keto or low-carb diet. The recipes will transform your former carb-loving self into a keto junk food connoisseur!

This chapter discusses the ketogenic diet, including what it is, the macronutrient breakdown, how to tell when your body switches over to using ketones for energy, and what to expect when your body is in ketosis. It will also go over keto cooking basics and explain some of the more unusual keto ingredients.

What Is the Keto Diet?

A keto diet is a low-carbohydrate, moderate-protein, high-fat diet. When you reduce your intake of carbohydrates (your body's usual source of energy), your body is forced to adapt and make ketones to use for energy instead. If you're at a caloric surplus, your body will use these ketones and fatty acid for fuel, but if you're at a caloric deficit, your body will tap into its fat storage and use your existing fat for fuel.

Let's talk about what happens in your body when you eat carbs. Carbohydrate digestion occurs in the gastrointestinal tract, starting in the mouth. First, your body breaks down the carbs into glucose, and then that glucose enters the bloodstream through the small intestines, causing blood glucose (blood sugar) to rise. This rise in blood sugar triggers insulin to transport glucose from your blood into your cells so it can be used as energy. When you eat more carbohydrates than your body needs for fuel, the excess is stored as fat in the form of triglycerides.

However, when your carb intake is limited, your body must turn to alternative fuel sources. First your body will use its stored glucose (called glycogen) from the muscle and liver. After that, it will break down fat for energy; that fat comes either from your diet or from stored fat in the form of fatty acids and ketones (also called ketone bodies). Even when your carb intake is limited, your body still runs on a combination of glucose, ketones, and fatty acids because your body continues to produce glucose through a process called gluconeogenesis. Because of this, carbs are not a required macronutrient for most people.

When transitioning into a ketogenic diet, the method of transition is largely based on each individual person. Some people do well going "cold turkey" and jumping right into a strict keto diet, while others need to gradually reduce their carbohydrate intake a few weeks prior to starting a ketogenic diet to be able to succeed. Additionally, a person's motivation for starting a ketogenic lifestyle plays a role. For example, if a doctor prescribes a keto diet for someone with epilepsy, they may start it sooner than someone who starts a keto diet for weight loss.

What Is Ketosis?

Ketosis is the state of having elevated blood ketone levels, meaning that your body is now effectively burning fat for energy instead of carbohydrates. This can happen a few different ways:

- *By following a very low-carb, high-fat diet*
- *By fasting (not eating or consuming drinks with calories)*
- *By prolonged strenuous exercise*

When you are in ketosis, your body produces ketones to use as fuel, either from the fat you eat or from the stored fat in your body. When you're in a state of nutritional ketosis, it's easier to tap into stored fat for fuel than if you were on a carbohydrate-based diet. This is because your blood sugar level isn't constantly being spiked due to carbohydrate intake; with more consistent blood sugar levels, you are less likely to have hunger pangs and cravings. Because fat is so satiating, it's easier to eat at a caloric deficit and not feel deprived.

When your body is already running on fat for fuel, it will more readily tap into stored fat. This is because insulin isn't constantly being secreted, so fat-burning mode is left on. When eating at a caloric deficit while following a ketogenic diet, weight loss occurs. A big benefit of a ketogenic diet for weight loss is that you preserve more lean body mass and lose a higher percentage of fat than you would on a higher-carb diet. Limiting carbohydrate intake forces your body to run on fat as your primary fuel source and puts you into a state of nutritional ketosis.

What Are Macronutrients?

Macronutrients include carbohydrates, protein, and fats. They're called macronutrients because they're typically consumed in large quantities and are measured in grams instead of micrograms or milligrams. Fat and protein are needed in large amounts to ensure that your body runs efficiently and to preserve lean body mass. Previously carbohydrates were thought to be required, but now we know that isn't the case for most people because of gluconeogenesis. All of the foods that you eat contain at least one macronutrient. Carbohydrates and protein contain 4 calories (kcals) per gram, while fat contains 9 calories (kcals) per gram. On a typical ketogenic diet, the macronutrient breakdown is as follows:

- *60–75 percent of calories from fat*
- *15–30 percent of calories from protein*
- *5–10 percent of calories from carbohydrates*

Signs You're in Ketosis

During the first two weeks of being on the keto diet you may experience some symptoms that people refer to as the "keto flu." These symptoms may consist of the following:

- *Headaches*
- *Chills*
- *Ashy skin tone*
- *Sensitivity to light and sound*
- *Nausea*
- *Dizziness*
- *Brain fog*
- *Insomnia*
- *Irritability*
- *GI issues*

Some people say that the keto flu is your body's way of telling you that you're going through carbohydrate withdrawal, and in a way, it is. These symptoms pass the way a normal flu would pass once your body adjusts to running on ketones, which can take anywhere from three days to two weeks.

There are a few things you can do to mitigate or speed up the symptoms of the keto flu:

- *Get plenty of electrolytes in the form of bone broth, pickle juice, and so on.*
- *Drink lots of water.*
- *Make sure to get enough sleep.*
- *If your doctor approves it, take magnesium and potassium supplements.*
- *Be patient with yourself—the brain fog will eventually go away and your productivity will increase.*

After you've gone through the keto flu period, the good stuff starts. Positive signs that you're in ketosis include:

- *Increased energy*
- *Increased focus*
- *Decreased appetite*
- *Improved mood*
- *Decreased inflammation*
- *Weight loss (if eating at a caloric deficit)*
- *Elevated blood ketone levels*

▶ Tools to Test for Ketones (in Breath, Urine, and Blood)

To be successful on the keto diet, you don't need to test yourself unless you're using this diet for therapeutic purposes or a doctor recommends it. For those who want to test, there are a few ways to test whether you're in a state of nutritional ketosis, and some are more accurate than others. When you first start a keto diet, you may not want to invest over $100 for a blood or breath meter, so you may opt for ketone urine test strips. These urine test strips are very inexpensive (under $10 for one hundred strips) and test for the presence of ketone bodies, specifically the ketone acetoacetate. These strips are an indicator that your body is now producing ketones, but currently your body is excreting them through the urine. This is the first sign you're on your way to becoming fat-adapted. This means your body is using fatty acids and ketones as a primary fuel source, which is the point of a ketogenic diet.

Once you have been following a keto diet for a while and are committed, you may decide to purchase a blood glucose meter and blood ketone meter. These meters measure blood levels of the ketone beta-hydroxybutyrate (BHB), along with blood glucose. The level of ketones in your blood indicates how deep a state of ketosis you're in. Ketones and glucose have an inverse relationship, meaning when ketone levels rise, blood sugar lowers. Some diseases or conditions that are treated with a ketogenic diet may require deeper states of ketosis to be therapeutic. The higher ketone levels are, the deeper the state of nutritional ketosis. Blood meters cost between $50 and $100, and are available online. We use the Keto-Mojo meter because at this time it's a fraction of the cost per strip of other brands. This meter is available on the *Keto-Mojo* website and elsewhere online.

If you have a little more money to spend, some people opt for getting a breath ketone meter. A couple popular brands are Ketonix and LEVL. The Ketonix meter costs in the range of $150 to $250 and is available for purchase on their website. The LEVL meter is only available through the company's website for a monthly fee, which starts at $99 per month. These meters measure the amount of acetone in the breath, which is formed from the breakdown of acetoacetate (a by-product of fat metabolism), indicating that you're burning fat.

(However, this doesn't necessarily mean that you're in ketosis. For example, after an intense workout it would show the presence of acetone in the breath because you're using fat for fuel during the workout, although you may not be in ketosis.)

Tips for Your Keto Journey

Because the keto diet can be tricky and very different from the standard American diet, here are a few tips to help you succeed:

- *Use keto junk food as a tool to help satisfy your carb cravings while maintaining nutritional ketosis.*

- *Eat a variety of foods, focusing on low-carb, high-fat options such as grass-fed meat and dairy; free-range chicken and eggs; wild-caught seafood; seeds and nuts; low-carb fruits such as berries, avocados, coconut, and olives; and low-carb vegetables such as leafy greens, cruciferous vegetables, and other nonstarchy vegetables.*

- *Choose top-quality healthy fats such as grass-fed lard or tallow, coconut oil, avocado oil, olive oil, grass-fed butter, and/or ghee.*

- *Eat foods high in magnesium and potassium or use supplements to make sure you're getting enough electrolytes to avoid muscle cramping. Similarly, make sure you're getting 3–5 grams of sodium per day (or follow your physician's advice on sodium intake) to keep your electrolyte levels balanced. We recommend using a high-quality sea salt like Redmond Real Salt, which is typically available online or in many grocery stores. Some people choose to use an electrolyte powder such as Dr. Berg's Electrolyte Powder or Vega Sport Hydrator.*

- *Stay hydrated—water is the best way to do this! A good rule is to consume half your body weight in pounds in ounces of water daily.*

- *Get into a routine where you're meal planning and meal prepping to save time and money, and to avoid having to resort to high-carb or fast food on busy days.*

Why You Should Make Keto Junk Food

You can use keto junk food as a tool to help you stay on track and stay in ketosis. In our culture, junk food is everywhere we look; we see ads for it on billboards, on TV, on social media, and more. There's no escaping it! But the things we think of as junk food don't have to be off-limits on the keto diet. Once you start making the recipes from this cookbook, it'll blow your mind with how close these keto versions of classic junk foods are to "regular" junk food items! We've found that anything you're craving from your pre-keto days can most likely be recreated in a low-carb, high-fat version of itself. Think of keto junk food as a way to nourish yourself with healthy energy sources without spiking your blood sugar levels, all while satisfying your cravings and enjoying the familiar most bad-for-you-sounding junky foods you love.

Keto junk food is a win-win.

The thing about a ketogenic diet, like any other diet where you're avoiding certain foods (here, it's carbs that are the devil…well, not really, but we tend to avoid them at all costs), is that it's a mental thing. If you tell yourself you can't have junk food, you'll want junk food even more. Let's give an example: Right now, don't imagine a red car. Whatever you do, don't picture a red car in your mind. You can think about baseball or a glass of milk, but just don't envision a red car! Okay, by now you're probably seeing nothing but a red car in your head. This is just the way our brains operate. If we're told that we can't do or can't have something, it's all we can think about and we want it way more than we normally would.

Junk food definitely has a negative connotation, especially for people starting a diet (even though we don't really like to think of a ketogenic lifestyle as a diet!). Many of us have the idea that junk food is bad and off-limits, and then throw into the mix the fact that you decided to go keto and you're learning the ins and outs of this way of eating. Then suddenly, even though you didn't even like junk food that much to begin with, junk food is now all you can think about.

If that sounds a little too familiar, this junk food cookbook will save you!

We made waffles that you'd swear are regular waffles (and are perfect for making into Savory BBQ Breakfast Waffles, Waffle Egg Sandwiches, and Ice Cream Sundae Waffles…or for freezing and eating on busy mornings!). Pizza Night is back in regular rotation, Meat Lover's Pizza included, as well as Chicken Nugs and Garlic Parmesan Wings. Or if you like the sweet and salty crunch of Asian takeout classics like General Tso's Chicken and Orange Chicken, we have you covered, and we even make a pretty mean Fried "Rice" or Keto Lo Mein to round out the meal. Of course, recipes for just about anything your kids could ask you to make for Taco Tuesday are in this book—Loaded Nachos, Taco Salad Bowls, and Tortilla Chips included. And yes, there is dessert! If you're a chocoholic you'll want to check out our Quadruple Chocolate Cake or Chocolate Overload Milkshake, but if vanilla is more your thing, take a look at our Basic Vanilla Cake, Vanilla Ice Cream, and Your Not-So-Basic Vanilla Shake. Because they're a quintessential part of junk food, we have a ton of cookies, candy, and other cakes as well.

This book will be your new best friend for turning a keto diet into a way of life, instead of just a diet.

Keto Baking Basics

Now that you know how useful keto junk food is to help you stay on track, let's talk about junk food, keto-style. Junk food on a keto diet is a whole new world! Bready and cakey high-carb items are a huge part of junk food, and when you're making junk food keto-friendly, there are no high-carb, gluten-filled flours to help bready and cakey items bind easily, such as wheat flour, cake flour, all-purpose flour, potato flour, quinoa flour, or brown rice flour. Instead, we typically use low-carb, high-fat ingredients like coconut flour, almond flour, sunflower seed flour, flaxseed meal, and other similar flours. Also, we use melted part-skim mozzarella cheese to make a delicious dough for things like pizza and breadsticks.

But what about binders and emulsifiers? In normal baking, gluten acts as a binder and creates a soft-textured product with a light crumb. However, with ketogenic baking, we don't use flour sources that contain gluten, so we have to improvise to get similar results. Psyllium husk, beef gelatin, ground flaxseeds, xanthan gum, and guar gum are commonly used in keto baking to help bind and emulsify baked goods.

And of course, keto baking doesn't use sugary items such as honey, maple syrup, brown sugar, white sugar, agave nectar, and so on. We opt for sugar substitutes that won't cause a blood sugar spike, like stevia, erythritol, monk fruit, and so on. Our favorite way to sweeten keto baked goods is with a combination of stevia and erythritol, because stevia helps reduce the cooling effect of erythritol, and erythritol helps cut the bitterness of stevia. (By cooling effect, we mean that erythritol can cause a cool breath feeling as if you just ate a mint, but without the minty flavor.)

Noodles are also a junk food staple, and we've become well versed in the world of low-carb and keto-friendly noodles! Spiralized zucchini is always a favorite, and we also love spiralized daikon radish, celeriac, and yellow summer squash. Ever since we discovered them, Palmini noodles (which are made from hearts of palm and are available in a can) have been one of our new favorites, and we use them to make Singapore Noodles, Keto Lo Mein, and Keto Pad Thai.

Let's not forget that a lot of the appeal of savory junk food is the crunch factor! Battered and fried, there's something about it that appeals to us. To replace regular bread crumbs, we love using almond flour, sometimes combined with coconut flour and/or Parmesan cheese and seasonings for a crisp coating.

Sometimes it takes a little creativity, but we've realized that just about any recipe can be made into a keto version of itself!

The Keto Pantry

A keto pantry looks nothing like your typical pantry! There are no boxed brownie or cookie mixes, canned or dried beans, boxes of Hamburger Helper or mac and cheese, canola oil, vegetable oil, salad dressings full of carbs and highly processed oil, cookies, rice, wheat flour, sugar, crackers, or candy.

On the other hand, a typical keto pantry might include the following:

- *Seeds and nuts such as sunflower seeds, pecans, Brazil nuts, macadamia nuts, walnuts, almonds, and pistachios*
- *Alternative flours like coconut flour, almond flour, and flaxseed meal*
- *Canned Palmini noodles*
- *Low-carb protein powders and collagen peptides*
- *Healthy fats, including coconut oil, avocado oil, olive oil, ghee, MCT oil, and MCT oil powder*
- *Nut butters such as almond butter, coconut butter or manna, cacao butter, peanut butter, or macadamia nut butter*
- *Snacks like low-sugar jerky, olives, unsweetened coconut chips, and dill pickles*
- *Condiments such as tamari sauce or coconut aminos, vinegars (like apple cider vinegar, red wine vinegar, and white wine vinegar), mustard, low-sugar ketchup and marinara sauce, dressings made with avocado oil, and mayonnaise made with avocado oil*
- *Dried spices and herbs*
- *Sugar alternatives such as stevia, erythritol, monk fruit, allulose, and so on*

As you can see, these two pantries are drastically different. The former is full of highly processed, highly refined foods that are mostly high in carbs and are hyperpalatable. Basically, they're made full of sugar and chemicals to taste really good. When you eat only from the former pantry, your taste buds get accustomed to supersweet foods. It takes some time, but you can retrain your palate.

Demystifying Keto Junk Food Staples

Keto junk food has some strange products that you may never have heard of before, so here is a brief description of some of the more common ingredients used.

▶ Pre-Shredded Low-Moisture Part-Skim Mozzarella Cheese

This product is probably familiar, but not in the way we use it! We melt it down and use it as the base for things like pizza and breadsticks. And yes, we're talking about the kind you find pre-shredded in the plastic bags at the grocery store, not the block of cheese you shred yourself.

▶ Coconut Flour

Coconut flour is made from dried ground coconut meat, and nowadays is readily available at most supermarkets. Coconut flour is both gluten-free and low in carbohydrates, which makes it a popular baking choice for the low-carb, Paleo, and gluten-free communities. It's very high in fiber compared with other flours, and you'll need much less of it compared to other flours, such as all-purpose flour in traditional baking or almond flour in low-carb baking.

Coconut flour can be a little finicky to work with. Note that if you are using coconut flour alone in baked goods, your breads and baked goods may turn out a little on the drier, denser side. This is most likely due to the high fiber content of coconut flour and the fact that it absorbs a lot of liquid. Baked goods recipes that use a lot of coconut flour tend to add a lot of eggs to help lighten, moisten, and bind the recipe, and to provide structure.

In addition to using coconut flour in keto baked goods, we like to use it in combination with almond flour as a replacement for regular bread crumbs.

▶ Almond Flour

Almond flour comes from raw almonds that have had their skins removed. It's not to be confused with almond meal, which is made from raw almonds that still have their skin on and is darker in color. Both almond flour and almond meal are used in keto baking.

Almond flour is naturally gluten-free and low in carbohydrates, and is often used in low-carb baking to replace traditional all-purpose flour. Almond flour is higher in fat and lower in fiber than coconut flour, and is normally used in higher amounts than coconut flour in recipes. Many keto and low-carb baking recipes call for a blend of both coconut and almond flour for the best results in terms of flavor and texture.

Keto baked goods that use almond flour often have psyllium husk powder, beef gelatin, and/or flaxseed meal added to them. This is to help provide a chewy bread-like texture and structure. In addition to using almond flour in keto baked goods, we like to use it in combination with coconut flour as a replacement for regular bread crumbs.

▶ Psyllium Husk Powder

This is a finely ground powder made of psyllium husks. It is very high in fiber and contains a lot of water. Psyllium husk powder is used to add a more bread-like texture to keto baked goods because of their lack of gluten. Make sure you check the label and get psyllium husk powder instead of psyllium husks because they aren't interchangeable. Also, note that depending on what brand of psyllium husk powder you use, it may turn your baked goods purplish or grayish in color; it shouldn't affect the flavor, though. We recommend using Bob's Red Mill Psyllium Fiber Powder or Viva Naturals Organic Psyllium Husk Powder, both of which are available online.

▶ Beef Gelatin

If you're familiar with gelatin desserts, you're already familiar with gelatin! In keto baking, beef gelatin helps achieve a chewy texture. As you'll see in the recipes in this book, a little goes a long way. Be sure to follow the recipe and dissolve the gelatin in boiling water before adding it to the batter or dough. Try grass-fed and pasture-raised beef gelatin for the most nutrition.

▶ Flaxseed Meal

Flaxseed meal is made by grinding up flaxseeds into a fine powder. There are two standard types, brown and golden. Both work interchangeably in recipes, but if you have a recipe that is a lighter color, using the golden flaxseed meal will make your recipe look prettier instead of having dark specks throughout the finished product. Flaxseeds are a good source of fiber and provide omega-3 fatty acids in the form of alpha-linolenic acid (ALA). Ground flaxseeds are also used in vegan baking to make a vegan egg replacement.

▶ Chia Seeds

Chia seeds can be used in baking either in their whole form or in a powdered form. To make powdered chia seeds, simply blend them in a high-speed blender until powdery. Chia seeds are great to add to recipes to absorb liquid and to give a chewier texture to keto baked goods. They are also high in fiber and protein with 0 grams of net carbs per serving, making them a great keto option.

▶ Stevia

This keto-friendly sweetener comes from the leaves of a plant. Stevia is used as a sugar substitute, but tastes much sweeter than cane sugar; it can be up to three hundred times as sweet! Some people note that stevia can have a bitter aftertaste. There are several forms of stevia available, such as liquid (usually comes with a dropper), stevia glycerite (which is more viscous than regular liquid stevia and even more highly concentrated), and powdered stevia. In its powdered form, stevia is commonly blended with another sweetener, such as erythritol, to reduce the bitterness. Be on the lookout for stevia blends that contain maltodextrin or dextrose, both of which contain calories and elicit an insulin and glucose response.

▶ Erythritol

Erythritol is very popular in keto and low-carb baking because of its very low glycemic index. Erythritol is not an artificial sweetener; rather, it's a sugar alcohol derived from corn or sugarcane. Erythritol typically comes in a granulated form like granulated sugar and a confectioners' or powdered form like powdered sugar. Erythritol contains about 0.25 kcals per gram; compare that with regular sugar, which contains 4 kcals per gram. Erythritol is only about 70 percent as sweet as sugar, so you will need to increase the amount when swapping it for sugar to achieve the same level of sweetness. But note, erythritol in higher quantities tends to create a cooling effect. Because of this, a lot of sweet baked goods recipes use a blend of erythritol and stevia to counteract both the cooling effect of erythritol and the bitter taste of stevia. Note that because erythritol is a sugar alcohol, some people may experience digestive issues if they consume it in large amounts.

▶ Monk Fruit

Native to China, monk fruit is another keto sweetener that's used as a sugar substitute. To make monk fruit sweetener, the fruit is dried and made into an extract, which is approximately 150 to 250 times as sweet as regular sugar. Monk fruit sweetener has no calories or carbs and doesn't impact blood glucose levels. You can find allulose–monk fruit and monk fruit–erythritol blends available on the market that mimic the sweetness of regular sugar.

▶ Allulose

Allulose is a gluten-free, low-calorie sweetener. It's found in small amounts in some foods, such as wheat, figs, and raisins. Allulose isn't metabolized by the body, so it doesn't cause blood sugar or insulin spikes. When it comes to taste and texture, allulose is very similar to regular sugar, although it's about 70 percent as sweet.

▶ Palmini Noodles

These plant-based noodles are made from the hearts of the palm plant and cut to look like different types of pasta, such as linguine noodles and lasagna noodles. They come in a can, and you can usually find them in the canned vegetable aisle at your regular grocery store.

Junk Food Without the Guilt

No matter what junk food used to be your go-to before going keto, we have something in this book you're going to love. We cover brunch, pizza night, burger joint and sub shop favorites, a bunch of Asian take-out dishes, taco night classics, bakery and ice cream shop treats, and even happy hour nibbles and drinks. The goal of this book is to teach you how to make fabulous keto junk foods so that you can enjoy the keto lifestyle without feeling deprived. This book will help you stay on track with your keto goals, and provide you with the recipes and knowledge to do so.

CHAPTER 2
Brunch Spot Favorites

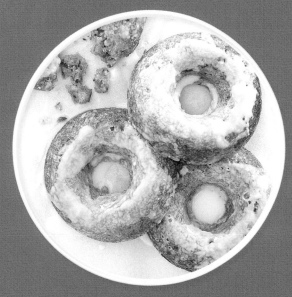

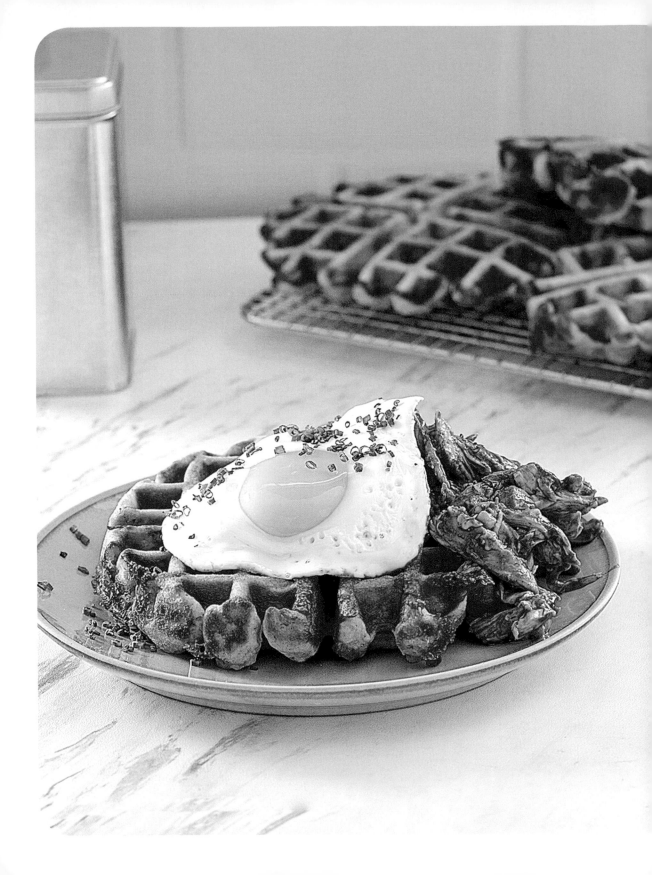

Savory BBQ Breakfast Waffles

With a blend of spices, as well as Cheddar cheese and fresh jalapeños, this waffle can serve double duty as a dinner biscuit with your favorite beanless chili. The jalapeños add nice flavor without too much heat; feel free to bump them up or omit them based on your preference.

SAVORY WAFFLES

4 tablespoons unsalted butter, melted and cooled slightly

6 ounces cream cheese, softened

4 large eggs

¾ cup almond flour

1 teaspoon psyllium husk powder

1 teaspoon baking powder

1 teaspoon onion powder

1 teaspoon garlic powder

1 teaspoon sweet paprika

¼ teaspoon ground black pepper

¼ teaspoon salt

3 tablespoons minced fresh jalapeños

1 cup shredded Cheddar cheese

Olive oil spray

OTHER

1 cup cooked, shredded chicken breast, heated

¼ cup Sweet BBQ Sauce (see Chapter 3)

4 large eggs, fried in 1 teaspoon avocado oil

4 teaspoons minced fresh chives

1 *For the Waffles:* In a medium bowl, whisk together butter, cream cheese, and eggs. Whisk in almond flour, psyllium husk powder, baking powder, onion powder, garlic powder, paprika, black pepper, and salt until combined. Stir in jalapeños and Cheddar. Let batter rest 2 minutes to thicken.

2 Plug in a waffle iron. Once heated, spray the inside with olive oil.

3 Pour ¼ of batter into the heated waffle iron and cook until waffle starts to steam, about 2–3 minutes. Carefully remove cooked waffle and cook remaining batter the same way.

4 *To Assemble:* In a small bowl, mix together shredded chicken and Sweet BBQ Sauce. Place one waffle on a plate. Top with ¼ of barbecue chicken, 1 fried egg, and 1 teaspoon chives. Repeat with remaining waffles. Serve warm.

Per Serving
Calories: 739 | Fat: 55g | Protein: 38g | Sodium: 890mg | Fiber: 3g | Carbohydrates: 19g | Net Carbohydrates: 8g | Sugar: 4g

Wow. This Tastes Like a Real Waffle. How Is That Possible?!

If you've been keto for a while and have tried your hand at baking, you probably know that it can be a challenge to replicate the results of gluten. Waffles should be crispy outside and tender inside with a bit of chew to them. Our keto waffles are similar thanks to psyllium husk powder for bready texture and shredded cheese for chewiness.

Cinnamon Bread

Nothing makes the house smell as much like a bakery as a loaf of Cinnamon Bread in the oven! We like ours with a schmear of cream cheese and fresh sliced strawberries or toasted with butter. Bake a loaf and use it to make Loaded French Toast and Cinnamon Bun Bread Pudding (see recipes in this chapter).

2 cups almond flour

2/3 cup granulated (or crystalized) allulose-monk fruit blend sweetener

1/2 cup golden flaxseed meal

2 tablespoons coconut flour

2 teaspoons ground cinnamon

3/4 teaspoon baking soda

3/4 teaspoon salt

1/2 teaspoon psyllium husk powder

6 large eggs

1/2 cup heavy whipping cream

1/4 cup water

1 tablespoon pure vanilla extract

1 1/2 teaspoons apple cider vinegar

1/4 teaspoon stevia glycerite

1/4 teaspoon butter extract

1 Preheat oven to 350°F. Line a 9" × 5" loaf pan with parchment paper.

2 In a large bowl, whisk together almond flour, allulose–monk fruit, flaxseed meal, coconut flour, cinnamon, baking soda, salt, and psyllium husk powder.

3 In a medium bowl, whisk together eggs, cream, water, vanilla, vinegar, stevia, and butter extract.

4 Add wet ingredients to dry ingredients and stir to combine, being careful not to overmix.

5 Pour batter into the prepared loaf pan and bake until a wooden skewer inserted in the center comes out clean, about 55–75 minutes. If necessary, cover the top with foil during the last 15 minutes of baking to prevent overbrowning.

6 Cool completely before slicing. Serve.

Per Serving (Serving size: 1 slice)
Calories: 236 | Fat: 19g | Protein: 9g | Sodium: 266mg | Fiber: 5g | Carbohydrates: 18g | Net Carbohydrates: 2g | Sugar: 2g

Loaded French Toast

In France, they call "French toast" pain perdu, *which translates to "lost bread." When you have bread (keto or otherwise) that's past its prime, what better use for it? Repurpose that lost bread into this delicious dish.*

FRENCH TOAST

1 large egg

2 tablespoons heavy whipping cream

1 tablespoon powdered erythritol

3 drops liquid stevia

½ teaspoon pure vanilla extract

½ teaspoon ground cinnamon

4 slices Cinnamon Bread (see recipe in this chapter)

1 tablespoon coconut oil

TOPPINGS

3 tablespoons heavy whipping cream, whipped to soft peaks

2 medium strawberries, thinly sliced

2 tablespoons fresh blueberries

2 tablespoons fresh raspberries

2 teaspoons stevia-sweetened mini chocolate chips

1 *For the French Toast:* In a shallow bowl, lightly beat together egg, cream, powdered erythritol, stevia, vanilla, and cinnamon. Dip each slice of bread in egg mixture, letting it soak in.

2 Heat a large nonstick skillet over medium heat. Once hot, add coconut oil. Once melted, add dipped bread slices.

3 Cook until the bread is golden on both sides, about 4–5 minutes on the first side and 2–3 minutes on the second side.

4 *To Serve:* Place two slices of French Toast each on two plates. Divide whipped cream, strawberries, blueberries, raspberries, and chocolate chips between them. Serve.

Per Serving
Calories: 728 | Fat: 61g | Protein: 22g | Sodium: 581mg | Fiber: 12g | Carbohydrates: 48g | Net Carbohydrates: 7g | Sugar: 6g

Chocolate Chip Pancakes

Nothing says Saturday morning breakfast better than pancakes. Well, maybe pancakes and fresh coffee. Whip these up and you're halfway there! Top with some fresh berries for extra sweetness. Just a heads-up: Leftover pancakes reheat well in the microwave.

3 tablespoons unsalted butter, melted

3 tablespoons granulated (or crystalized) allulose–monk fruit blend sweetener

2 large eggs

1½ teaspoons pure vanilla extract

½ cup almond flour

1 tablespoon golden flaxseed meal

1 teaspoon baking powder

½ teaspoon psyllium husk powder

⅛ teaspoon salt

1/16 teaspoon ground cinnamon

4 tablespoons stevia-sweetened chocolate chips

1 In a medium bowl, whisk together butter and allulose–monk fruit, and then whisk in eggs and vanilla.

2 Next, whisk in almond flour, flaxseed meal, baking powder, psyllium husk powder, salt, and cinnamon. Stir in chocolate chips.

3 Preheat a large nonstick skillet over medium-low heat. Once hot, add ¼ of batter (about ⅓ cup of batter) to skillet. Cook until golden on the first side (about 3 minutes), and then flip the pancake with a thin metal spatula and cook until golden on the second side (about 1–2 minutes). Repeat with remaining batter. Serve warm.

Per Serving
Calories: 532 | Fat: 46g | Protein: 15g | Sodium: 461mg | Fiber: 12g | Carbohydrates: 44g | Net Carbohydrates: 14g | Sugar: 2g | Sugar Alcohol: 6g

Customize Your Pancakes

Feel free to make these pancakes your own. We used chocolate chips here, but shredded coconut (2 tablespoons) or fresh blueberries (6 tablespoons) will also create pancake perfection.

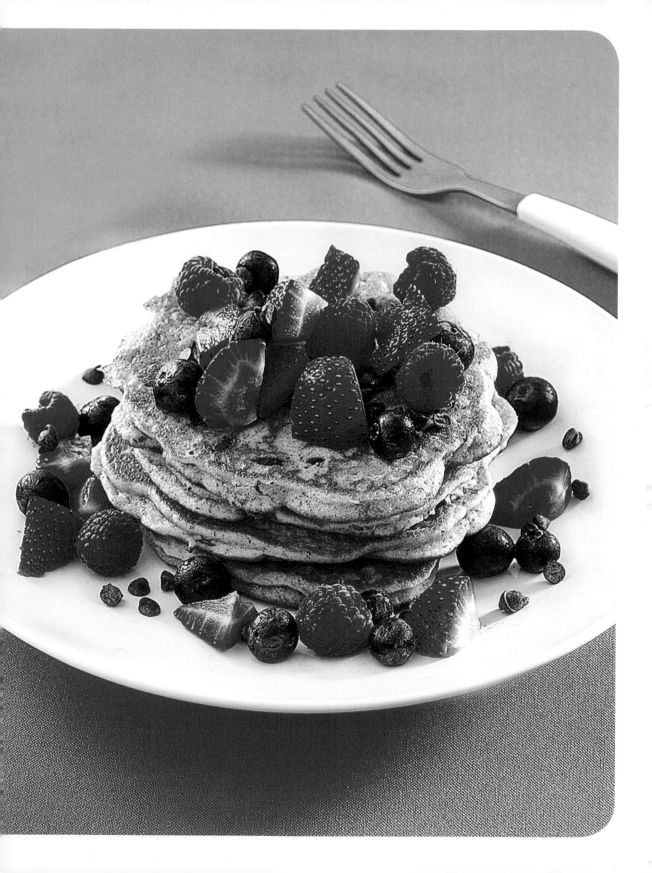

Cinnamon Bun Bread Pudding

Bread pudding is the perfect way to feed a crowd either breakfast or dessert with minimal effort. We use our Cinnamon Bread in this recipe, but feel free to swap it out for your favorite keto bread as long as the bread doesn't have savory flavor built in.

BREAD PUDDING

1 tablespoon unsalted butter, at room temperature
10 large egg yolks
1½ cups half and half
½ cup heavy whipping cream
⅓ cup granulated erythritol
20 drops liquid stevia
1 tablespoon pure vanilla extract
1 tablespoon ground cinnamon
¼ teaspoon salt
½ loaf Cinnamon Bread, cubed (see recipe in this chapter)

FROSTING

1½ cups heavy whipping cream
6 tablespoons unsalted butter
3 tablespoons Swerve Confectioners
20 drops liquid stevia
1/16 teaspoon salt
1 teaspoon pure vanilla extract

1 *For the Bread Pudding:* Smear butter on the inside of a 1½-quart casserole dish.

2 In a large bowl, beat egg yolks, half and half, cream, granulated erythritol, stevia, vanilla, cinnamon, and salt together. Add bread cubes and toss gently to coat.

3 Pour mixture into the prepared casserole dish, lightly pushing down on bread so it's mostly submerged in the liquid. Cover dish with foil and refrigerate overnight.

4 Preheat oven to 375°F. Get the casserole dish out of refrigerator and let it sit at room temperature 20 minutes while the oven preheats.

5 Bake casserole (covered with foil) 50 minutes, and then remove the foil and bake 5 minutes to lightly brown the top.

6 *For the Frosting:* To a medium saucepan over medium heat, add cream, butter, Swerve Confectioners, stevia, and salt.

7 Bring to a boil, and then cook until thickened to the consistency of melted frosting, about 12–15 minutes. It will thicken more as it cools, so don't overcook it.

8 Remove from heat and stir in vanilla.

9 *To Serve:* While bread pudding and frosting are both still hot, pour frosting on top of the pudding. Serve warm.

Per Serving
Calories: 485 | Fat: 44g | Protein: 10g | Sodium: 274mg | Fiber: 3g | Carbohydrates: 24g | Net Carbohydrates: 5g | Sugar: 4g

SERVES

10,

YIELDS 10
BUNS AND
18 TABLE-
SPOONS
FROSTING

Cinnamon Buns

For anyone who's ever walked past Cinnabon in the mall or airport and been tempted, we dedicate this recipe to you. Those sugar- and carb-heavy buns always leave us thinking that they smell better than they taste. That's not the case with this keto version! They have good bready texture, a rich cinnamon butter swirl, and a generous drizzle of frosting. If you like your buns on the gooey side, stay closer to the 20-minute cooking time.

FROSTING

1½ cups heavy whipping cream

6 tablespoons unsalted butter

3 tablespoons Swerve Confectioners

20 drops liquid stevia

1/16 teaspoon salt

1 teaspoon pure vanilla extract

FILLING

4 tablespoons unsalted butter, at room temperature

3 tablespoons keto brown sugar

1 tablespoon ground cinnamon

1 teaspoon pure vanilla extract

10 drops liquid stevia

DOUGH

Coconut oil spray

1 teaspoon instant yeast

2 tablespoons warm water

1¼ cups almond flour

2 tablespoons powdered allulose sweetener

Ingredients continued on the next page ▶

1 *For the Frosting:* To a medium saucepan over medium heat, add cream, butter, Swerve Confectioners, stevia, and salt.

2 Bring to a boil, and then cook until thickened to consistency of melted frosting, about 12–15 minutes. It will thicken more as it cools, so don't overcook it.

3 Remove from heat and stir in vanilla. Set aside.

4 *For the Filling:* In a small bowl, mix together all ingredients until well combined.

5 *For the Dough:* Preheat oven to 375°F. Spray the inside of a freezer- and oven-safe 9" pie plate or an 8" × 8" casserole dish with coconut oil.

6 In a small bowl, add yeast and warm water and stir to combine. Set aside until foamy, about 5–10 minutes.

7 In a medium bowl, whisk together almond flour, powdered allulose, psyllium husk powder, and baking powder and set aside.

8 In a large microwave-safe bowl, add mozzarella and cream cheese. Microwave 60 seconds and then give it a stir, and continue microwaving in 20-second increments until cheese is fully melted and combined when stirred.

Continued on the next page ▶

1¼ teaspoons psyllium husk powder

1 teaspoon baking powder

1½ cups pre-shredded low-moisture part-skim mozzarella

1 ounce cream cheese

1 large egg, lightly beaten

2 teaspoons pure vanilla extract

10 drops liquid stevia

½ tablespoon avocado oil, for oiling your hands

9 Stir yeast mixture into melted cheese until combined, and then stir in beaten egg, vanilla, and stevia until combined. Stir in almond flour mixture until it forms a shaggy dough.

10 Oil your hands and knead dough a couple times until it comes together as a ball.

11 Roll dough out between two pieces of parchment paper sprayed with coconut oil to a rectangle about 11" × 13".

12 Spread out cinnamon bun filling onto dough, leaving a border of about ¼" all the way around.

13 Starting with one of the short sides, tightly roll dough into a log. Cut log crosswise into ten equal pieces (each will be about 1"). Place rolls into the prepared dish and put in freezer to chill 10 minutes.

14 Transfer to oven and bake until rolls are golden, about 20–25 minutes.

15 *To Serve:* Serve cinnamon buns warm with about 1 tablespoon plus 2 teaspoons of frosting drizzled on top of each.

Per Serving

Calories: 391 | Fat: 35g | Protein: 9g | Sodium: 162mg | Fiber: 2g | Carbohydrates: 14g | Net Carbohydrates: 3g | Sugar: 2g | Sugar Alcohol: 7g

Waffle Egg Sandwiches

Crispy bacon, runny eggs, and Cheddar cheese sandwiched in a sweet waffle… there's no better way to start the day! We take that back. Serve up these Waffle Egg Sandwiches with a little keto-friendly maple-style syrup for dipping. That's even better.

SWEET WAFFLES

4 tablespoons unsalted butter, melted and cooled slightly

6 ounces cream cheese, softened

4 large eggs

1 tablespoon pure vanilla extract

¾ cup almond flour

¼ cup granulated (or crystalized) allulose sweetener

1 teaspoon psyllium husk powder

1 teaspoon baking powder

¼ teaspoon salt

1 cup pre-shredded low-moisture part-skim mozzarella cheese

Coconut oil spray

OTHER

4 large eggs, fried in 1 teaspoon avocado oil

2 (1-ounce) slices Cheddar cheese, cut in half

4 slices beef bacon, cooked until crispy

1 *For the Sweet Waffles:* In a large bowl, whisk together butter, cream cheese, eggs, and vanilla. Whisk in almond flour, allulose, psyllium husk powder, baking powder, and salt until combined. Stir in mozzarella. Let batter rest 2 minutes to thicken.

2 Plug in a waffle iron. Once heated, spray the inside with coconut oil.

3 Pour ¼ of batter into the heated waffle iron and cook until waffle starts to steam, about 2–3 minutes. Carefully remove cooked waffle and cook remaining batter the same way.

4 *To Make the Sandwiches:* Cut each waffle in half. Place one waffle half on a plate. Top with 1 fried egg, ½ slice cheese, and 1 slice bacon. Put the other half of waffle on top to make a sandwich. Repeat three times. Serve warm.

Per Serving
Calories: 800 | Fat: 63g | Protein: 35g | Sodium: 1,138mg | Fiber: 2g | Carbohydrates: 21g | Net Carbohydrates: 7g | Sugar: 4g

You Don't Like the Sweet and Savory Combo?

Instead of the Sweet Waffles for this recipe, make a batch of Savory Waffles from the Savory BBQ Breakfast Waffles recipe in this chapter and assemble as directed.

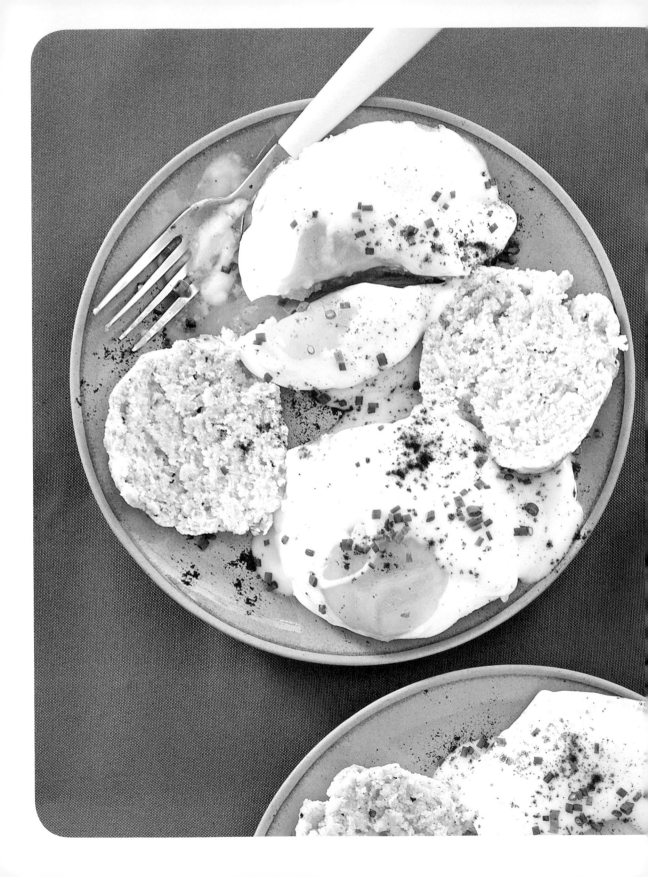

Biscuit Eggs Benedict

Eggs Benedict is one of those iconic brunch dishes that feels completely luxurious. This keto version features our favorite (easy!) homemade biscuits with a delicious blender hollandaise sauce and fried eggs. Smoky flavor comes from a sprinkle of smoked paprika, and chives add a pop of flavor and color.

BISCUITS

1 cup almond flour

1 teaspoon baking powder

$\frac{1}{4}$ teaspoon salt

$\frac{1}{8}$ teaspoon ground black pepper

2 tablespoons chilled unsalted butter, diced

2 tablespoons heavy whipping cream

1 large egg

$\frac{1}{2}$ cup shredded sharp white Cheddar cheese

BLENDER HOLLANDAISE SAUCE

2 large egg yolks

$\frac{1}{2}$ tablespoon fresh lemon juice

$\frac{1}{4}$ teaspoon Dijon mustard

$\frac{1}{8}$ teaspoon salt

$\frac{1}{16}$ teaspoon ground black pepper

5 tablespoons unsalted butter, melted and hot but not boiling

OTHER

4 large eggs, fried in 1 tablespoon avocado oil

2 teaspoons minced fresh chives

$\frac{1}{8}$ teaspoon smoked paprika

1 *For the Biscuits:* Preheat oven to 350°F. Line a baking sheet with a Silpat liner or parchment paper.

2 In a large bowl, use a fork to stir together almond flour, baking powder, salt, and black pepper. Cut in butter until it looks crumbly.

3 In a small bowl, beat together cream and egg, and gradually incorporate that into almond flour mixture. Stir in Cheddar until it's incorporated into dough.

4 Divide dough into four equal pieces and roll each into a ball (their shape doesn't have to be perfect). Arrange balls of dough on the prepared sheet and bake until golden on the bottom, about 20 minutes.

5 *For the Blender Hollandaise Sauce:* To a food processor, add egg yolks, lemon juice, Dijon, salt, and black pepper and process until smooth, about 1 minute, scraping down the sides as necessary.

6 Starting with one drop at a time, drizzle hot melted butter into egg yolk mixture with the motor running. Continue this way until half the butter is incorporated, and then add rest of butter in a slow, steady drizzle with the food processor running. You should end up with a smooth, emulsified sauce. If the sauce is too thick, drizzle water in ($\frac{1}{4}$ teaspoon at a time) until it reaches the right consistency.

Continued on the next page ▶

7 *To Assemble:* Split each biscuit in half and place the halves (cut side up) next to each other on each of four plates. Top each biscuit pair with 1 fried egg, ¼ of Blender Hollandaise Sauce (a scant 2 tablespoons each), ½ teaspoon minced fresh chives, and a sprinkle of smoked paprika.

8 Serve immediately.

Per Serving
Calories: 577 | Fat: 50g | Protein: 19g | Sodium: 560mg | Fiber: 3g | Carbohydrates: 7g | Net Carbohydrates: 4g | Sugar: 2g

Can You Make Hollandaise Sauce Ahead of Time?

We completely get it. We wanted to do this too. But let us ask you something: Would you make scrambled eggs ahead of time? Sadly, we wouldn't either. The same thing goes for hollandaise. Although you may be able to get it back to a pourable sauce-like consistency by reheating hollandaise in a double boiler, it just isn't the same.

Cheesy Bacon and Egg Breakfast Wraps

Here's a protein-rich breakfast idea that's just a little bit different from your standard bacon and egg breakfast. Feel free to customize the flavor profile by switching up the type of cheese and using any herbs or spices you like.

1 tablespoon salted butter

6 large eggs, lightly beaten

½ cup shredded Cheddar cheese

2 teaspoons minced fresh chives

⅛ teaspoon ground black pepper

4 (6"-8") low-carb tortilla wraps

8 slices beef bacon, cooked until crispy

1 Melt butter in a large nonstick skillet over medium heat. Add eggs and cook, stirring occasionally, until they're just barely set. Remove from heat.

2 Sprinkle Cheddar, chives, and black pepper on top. Drape a piece of foil on top of eggs until cheese is melted.

3 Evenly divide cheesy egg mixture between tortillas. Top each with 2 slices bacon. Serve.

Per Serving
Calories: 439 | Fat: 33g | Protein: 27g | Sodium: 1,007mg | Fiber: 11g | Carbohydrates: 16g | Net Carbohydrates: 5g | Sugar: 0g

Let's Do Breakfast Tomorrow!

This recipe is a great one to make ahead and stash in the refrigerator or freezer for a quick breakfast on the go. If you make them ahead, we recommend folding up these wraps like a burrito: Tuck in two opposite ends of a wrap, roll it up, and wrap it in parchment paper. These will last 3 days in the refrigerator or 3 months in the freezer, and you can reheat them in the microwave. (If they're coming out of the freezer, thaw them before reheating.)

Glazed Sour Cream Doughnuts

If cake-like sour cream doughnuts are your thing, then you're about to be a pretty happy camper! We keto-fied that classic, glaze and all. Paired with a hot cup of coffee, this makes a perfect weekend breakfast.

DOUGHNUTS

Coconut oil spray

2 tablespoons unsalted butter, slightly softened

¼ cup full-fat sour cream

3 tablespoons granulated (or crystalized) allulose sweetener

1 large egg

1 teaspoon pure vanilla extract

⅛ teaspoon almond extract

½ cup almond flour

1 tablespoon golden flaxseed meal

¾ teaspoon baking powder

½ teaspoon psyllium husk powder

⅛ teaspoon salt

¹⁄₁₆ teaspoon ground cinnamon

GLAZE

¼ cup powdered erythritol

½ teaspoon fresh lemon juice

½ teaspoon vanilla bean paste

¹⁄₁₆ teaspoon salt

4 teaspoons water

1 *For the Doughnuts:* Preheat oven to 350°F. Spray four wells of a doughnut pan with coconut oil.

2 In a large bowl, whisk together butter, sour cream, allulose, egg, vanilla, and almond extract. Add almond flour, flaxseed meal, baking powder, psyllium husk powder, salt, and cinnamon and whisk to combine.

3 Immediately pour batter into prepared wells of doughnut pan and tap pan down to help batter spread out in the wells. Let pan rest 3 minutes for batter to thicken.

4 Bake 15–17 minutes until doughnuts are golden and a toothpick inserted in the center comes out clean.

5 Let doughnuts cool in the pan for a couple minutes, then turn them out onto a wire rack to cool completely.

6 *For the Glaze:* Once doughnuts are cooled, whisk together all glaze ingredients in a small bowl.

7 Dip the top of each doughnut in glaze and then return doughnuts to a wire rack for glaze to set. Let glaze harden before serving.

Per Serving
Calories: 202 | Fat: 17g | Protein: 5g | Sodium: 225mg | Fiber: 2g | Carbohydrates: 22g | Net Carbohydrates: 2g | Sugar: 1g | Sugar Alcohol: 9g

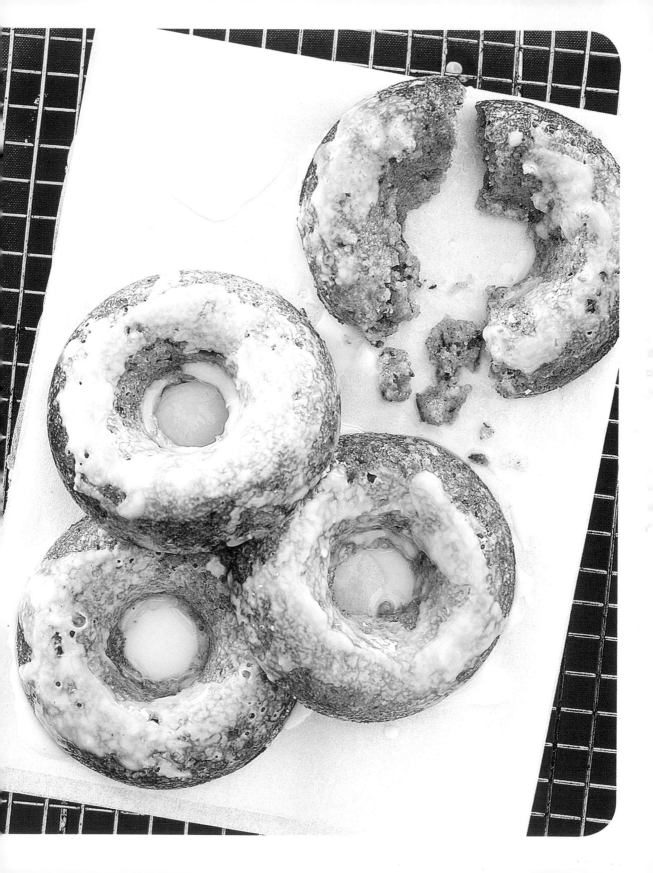

Strawberry Shortcake Doughnuts

In Buffalo, New York, there's a local institution called Paula's Donuts. They make the best melt-in-your-mouth doughnuts in the best flavors that you'll ever eat! Paula's Donuts' Strawberry Shortcake Doughnut with strawberry jam and vanilla buttercream was our inspiration for this.

DOUGHNUTS

Coconut oil spray

2 tablespoons unsalted butter, slightly softened

¼ cup full-fat sour cream

3 tablespoons granulated (or crystalized) allulose sweetener

1 large egg

1 teaspoon pure vanilla extract

⅛ teaspoon almond extract

½ cup almond flour

1 tablespoon golden flaxseed meal

¾ teaspoon baking powder

½ teaspoon psyllium husk powder

⅛ teaspoon salt

¹⁄₁₆ teaspoon ground cinnamon

OTHER

½ cup Basic Buttercream (see Chapter 7)

½ cup Strawberry Jam (see Chapter 7, part of the Strawberry Shortcake Cake Roll recipe)

1 *For the Doughnuts:* Preheat oven to 350°F. Spray four wells of a doughnut pan with coconut oil.

2 In a large bowl, whisk together butter, sour cream, allulose, egg, vanilla, and almond extract. Add almond flour, flaxseed meal, baking powder, psyllium husk powder, salt, and cinnamon and whisk to combine.

3 Immediately pour batter into prepared wells of doughnut pan and tap the pan down to help batter spread out in the wells. Let pan rest 3 minutes for batter to thicken.

4 Bake until doughnuts are golden and a toothpick inserted in the center comes out clean, about 15–17 minutes.

5 Let doughnuts cool in the pan for a couple minutes, then turn them out onto a wire rack to cool completely.

6 *To Assemble:* Spread 2 tablespoons of Basic Buttercream on top of each doughnut.

7 Spread 2 tablespoons of Strawberry Jam on top of Buttercream on each doughnut. Serve.

Per Serving
Calories: 276 | Fat: 23g | Protein: 6g | Sodium: 233mg | Fiber: 3g | Carbohydrates: 42g | Net Carbohydrates: 4g | Sugar: 4g

CHAPTER 3

Pizza Night

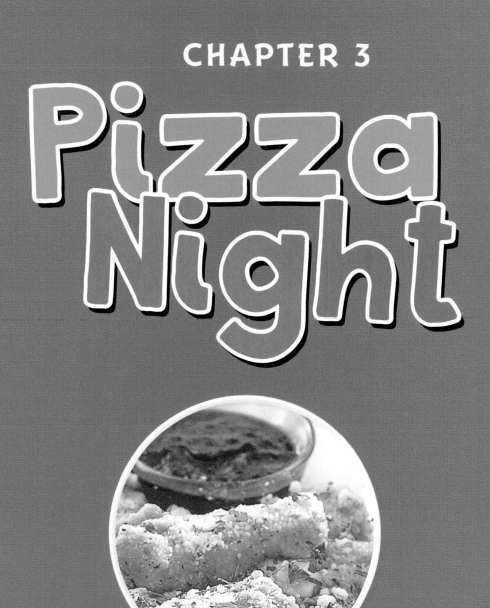

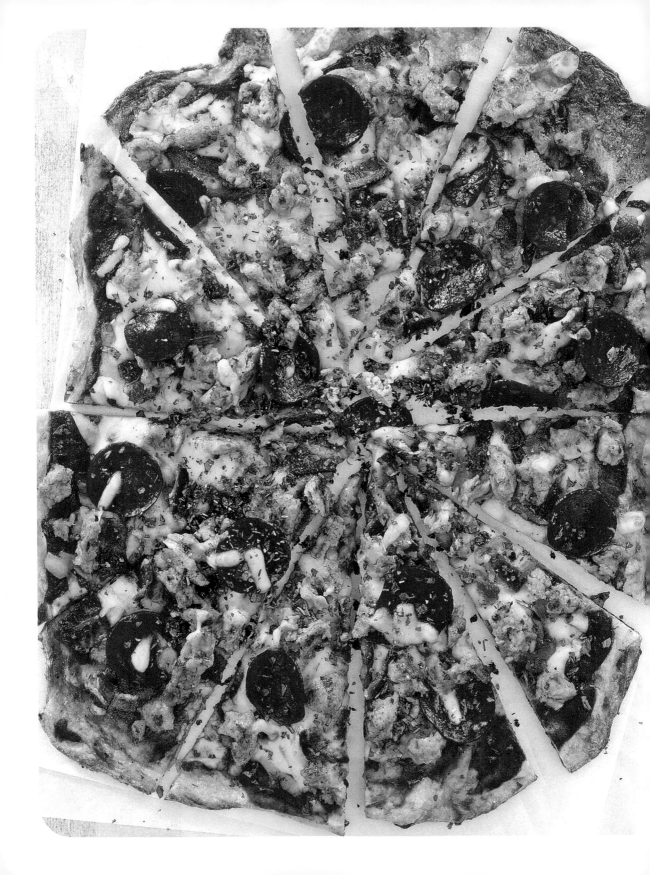

Meat Lover's Pizza

With three kinds of meat and two kinds of cheese, this Meat Lover's Pizza is packed with protein and sure to satisfy! Be sure to look for no-sugar-added pizza sauce so you're not adding hidden carbs to your pizza in the form of sugary tomato sauce.

PIZZA DOUGH

1 teaspoon instant yeast

2 tablespoons warm water

1 cup almond flour

1 teaspoon psyllium husk powder

1 teaspoon baking powder

1½ cups pre-shredded low-moisture part-skim mozzarella

1 ounce cream cheese

1 large egg, lightly beaten

½ tablespoon avocado oil, for oiling your hands

PIZZA TOPPINGS

¾ cup no-sugar-added pizza sauce

6 ounces shredded full-fat mozzarella cheese

2 ounces shredded sharp white Cheddar cheese

½ pound mild Italian turkey sausage crumbles, browned

4 slices beef bacon, cooked until crispy, and then crumbled

16 slices turkey pepperoni

1 teaspoon dried Italian herb seasoning

1 *For the Pizza Dough:* Preheat oven to 425°F. If you have a clay baking stone, place it in the center of the oven to preheat.

2 In a small bowl, add yeast and warm water and stir to combine. Set aside until foamy, about 5–10 minutes.

3 In a medium bowl, whisk together almond flour, psyllium husk powder, and baking powder and set aside.

4 In a large microwave-safe bowl, add mozzarella and cream cheese. Microwave 60 seconds and then give it a stir, and continue microwaving in 20-second increments until cheese is fully melted and combined when stirred.

5 Stir yeast mixture into melted cheese until combined, and then stir in beaten egg until combined. Stir in almond flour mixture until it forms a dough.

6 Oil your hands and knead dough a couple times until it comes together as a ball.

7 Roll out dough between two pieces of parchment paper to a 12" circle. Poke dough in several places with a fork.

8 Slide dough onto the preheated clay baking stone and bake until it's starting to turn golden brown in spots, about 6 minutes. If using a baking sheet instead of a clay baking stone, cook 8 minutes.

Continued on the next page ▶

9 *To Assemble and Bake the Pizza:* Once crust is prebaked, spread pizza sauce on top. Sprinkle on ¾ of mozzarella and Cheddar cheeses, reserving ¼ for topping. Spread browned sausage, crumbled bacon, pepperoni, remaining mozzarella and Cheddar cheeses, and Italian herb seasoning on top.

10 Return pizza to oven and bake until cheese is melted, about 10–15 minutes. Serve.

Per Serving
Calories: 390 | Fat: 27g | Protein: 24g | Sodium: 942mg | Fiber: 2g | Carbohydrates: 9g | Net Carbohydrates: 7g | Sugar: 3g

Can You Use Pork Sausage Instead of Turkey Sausage?

Yes! Once the pork sausage is browned, drain off any fat because it typically has a higher fat content than turkey sausage and we don't want the extra grease to make the pizza soggy. Note that using a different kind of sausage will change the nutritional information for this recipe.

BBQ Chicken Pizza

Before going keto, frozen BBQ chicken pizza was a staple in our freezer. If BBQ chicken pizza was your thing, too, this keto version of that classic flavor combo will take you back!

PIZZA DOUGH

1 teaspoon instant yeast

2 tablespoons warm water

1 cup almond flour

1 teaspoon psyllium husk powder

1 teaspoon baking powder

1½ cups pre-shredded low-moisture part-skim mozzarella

1 ounce cream cheese

1 large egg, lightly beaten

½ tablespoon avocado oil, for oiling your hands

PIZZA TOPPINGS

½ cup Sweet BBQ Sauce (see recipe in this chapter)

4 ounces shredded full-fat mozzarella cheese

4 ounces shredded sharp white Cheddar cheese

1 cup shredded, cooked chicken breast

4 slices beef bacon, cooked until crispy, and then crumbled

1 medium scallion, green and white parts, thinly sliced

3 tablespoons chopped fresh cilantro, for garnish

1 *For the Pizza Dough:* Preheat oven to 425°F. If you have a clay baking stone, place it in the center of the oven to preheat.

2 In a small bowl, add yeast and warm water and stir to combine. Set aside until foamy, about 5–10 minutes.

3 In a medium bowl, whisk together almond flour, psyllium husk powder, and baking powder and set aside.

4 In a large microwave-safe bowl, add mozzarella and cream cheese. Microwave 60 seconds and then give it a stir, and continue microwaving in 20-second increments until cheese is fully melted and combined when stirred.

5 Stir yeast mixture into melted cheese until combined, and then stir in beaten egg until combined. Stir in almond flour mixture until it forms a dough.

6 Oil your hands and knead dough a couple times until it comes together as a ball.

7 Roll out dough between two pieces of parchment paper to a 12" circle. Poke dough in several places with a fork.

8 Slide dough circle onto the preheated clay baking stone and bake until it's starting to turn golden brown in spots, about 6 minutes. If using a baking sheet instead of a clay baking stone, cook 8 minutes.

Continued on the next page ▶

9   *To Assemble and Bake the Pizza:* Once crust is prebaked, spread Sweet BBQ Sauce on top. Sprinkle on ¾ of mozzarella and Cheddar cheeses, reserving ¼ for topping. Spread chicken, bacon, scallion, and remaining mozzarella and Cheddar cheeses on top.

10 Return pizza to oven and bake until the cheese is melted, about 10–15 minutes.

11 Sprinkle cilantro on top and serve.

Per Serving
Calories: 369 | Fat: 25g | Protein: 24g | Sodium: 645mg | Fiber: 2g | Carbohydrates: 15g | Net Carbohydrates: 5g | Sugar: 3g

Triple Cheese Pizza

If you like plain cheese pizza (where are our Home Alone *fans?), you're going to go crazy for this Triple Cheese Pizza! A combination of mozzarella, fontina, and sharp white Cheddar makes this an ultra-cheesy, ultra-flavorful pizza. Pro tip: Sprinkle a few fresh basil leaves on right before serving!*

PIZZA DOUGH

1 teaspoon instant yeast

2 tablespoons warm water

1 cup almond flour

1 teaspoon psyllium husk powder

1 teaspoon baking powder

1½ cups pre-shredded low-moisture part-skim mozzarella

1 ounce cream cheese

1 large egg, lightly beaten

½ tablespoon avocado oil, for oiling your hands

PIZZA TOPPINGS

¾ cup no-sugar-added pizza sauce

4 ounces shredded full-fat mozzarella cheese

2 ounces shredded fontina cheese

2 ounces shredded sharp white Cheddar cheese

Per Serving
Calories: 292 | Fat: 21g |
Protein: 16g | Sodium: 512mg |
Fiber: 2g | Carbohydrates: 7g |
Net Carbohydrates: 5g | Sugar: 2g

1 *For the Pizza Dough:* Preheat oven to 425°F. If you have a clay baking stone, place it in the center of the oven to preheat.

2 In a small bowl, add yeast and warm water and stir to combine. Set aside until foamy, about 5–10 minutes.

3 In a medium bowl, whisk together almond flour, psyllium husk powder, and baking powder and set aside.

4 In a large microwave-safe bowl, add mozzarella and cream cheese. Microwave 60 seconds and then give it a stir, and continue microwaving in 20-second increments until cheese is fully melted and combined when stirred.

5 Stir yeast mixture into melted cheese until combined, and then stir in beaten egg until combined. Stir in almond flour mixture until it forms a dough.

6 Oil your hands and knead dough a couple times until it comes together as a ball.

7 Roll dough out between two pieces of parchment paper to a 12" circle. Poke dough in several places with a fork.

8 Slide dough circle onto preheated clay baking stone and bake until it's starting to turn golden brown in spots, about 6 minutes. If using a baking sheet instead of a clay baking stone, cook 8 minutes.

9 *To Assemble and Bake the Pizza:* Once crust is prebaked, spread pizza sauce on top. Sprinkle on mozzarella, fontina, and Cheddar cheeses.

10 Return pizza to oven and bake until the cheese is melted, about 6–8 minutes. Serve.

Mozzarella Sticks

Gooey melted cheese inside and crispy seasoned breading outside, these Mozzarella Sticks are everything you're looking for in a pizzeria snack! Serve them up with no-sugar-added marinara sauce for dipping if desired. For this recipe, be sure to use pre-grated store-bought Parmesan cheese that comes in a plastic shaker-top can, not fresh-grated Parmesan cheese.

½ cup almond flour

½ cup pre-grated Parmesan cheese

½ tablespoon dried Italian herb seasoning

1 teaspoon onion powder

1 teaspoon garlic powder

½ teaspoon salt

¼ teaspoon ground black pepper

2 large eggs

1 tablespoon water

8 mozzarella cheese sticks, cut in half horizontally

½ tablespoon coconut flour

2 tablespoons olive oil

1 In a shallow bowl, whisk together almond flour, Parmesan, Italian herb seasoning, onion powder, garlic powder, salt, and black pepper.

2 Crack eggs into a second shallow bowl and lightly beat them with water.

3 To a gallon-sized zip-top plastic bag, add halved cheese sticks and coconut flour and shake to coat the cheese.

4 Shake off excess flour from a cheese stick, dip it in egg, and then dip it in almond flour mixture to coat, and place it on a large baking sheet. Continue until all the cheese sticks are breaded.

5 Place cheese sticks into the freezer, and freeze until solid, about 1–2 hours. Meanwhile, preheat oven to 400°F.

6 Remove cheese sticks from freezer and drizzle oil on top, rolling them around gently to coat.

7 Bake until cheese sticks are golden on both sides, about 7–10 minutes, flipping once halfway through the cooking time. Serve warm.

Per Serving
Calories: 368 | Fat: 28g | Protein: 21g | Sodium: 884mg | Fiber: 2g | Carbohydrates: 6g | Net Carbohydrates: 4g | Sugar: 1g

Can You Fry These Mozzarella Cheese Sticks?

Yes! To fry these instead of baking them, omit the olive oil drizzled on top. Instead, add 2" of avocado oil to the bottom of a 5-quart pot. Heat the oil over medium-high heat until it reaches 365°F. Carefully add half of the frozen breaded Mozzarella Sticks and fry until golden, about 1 minute. Fry the remaining frozen breaded Mozzarella Sticks the same way.

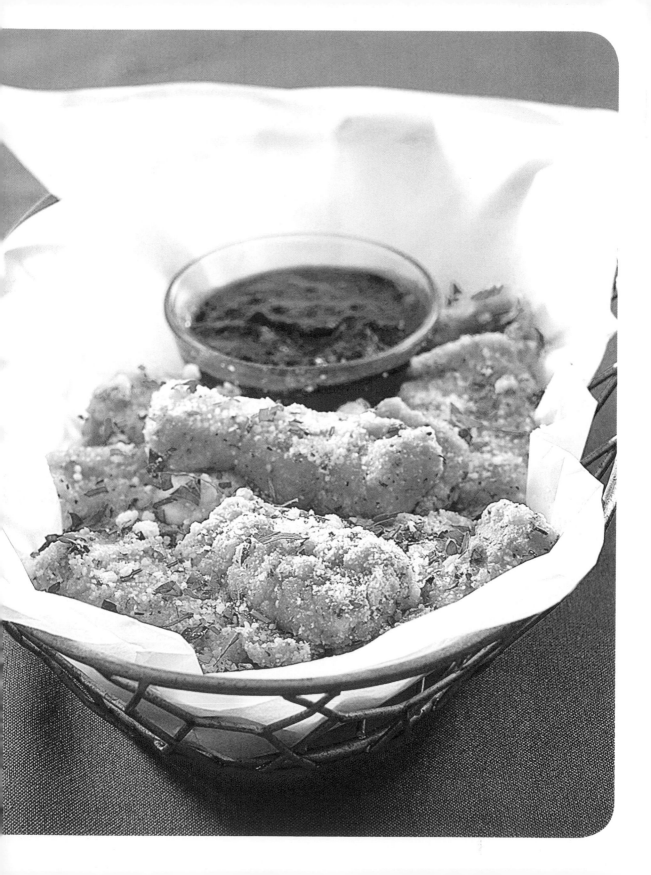

Garlic Breadsticks

Garlic Breadsticks are always a good idea. Pair them with an Italian dinner (low-carb pasta with tomato sauce, anyone?) or a meal of appetizers! We like to serve them with sugar-free marinara sauce for dipping. And if you want to add a handful of shredded mozzarella along with the garlic butter to turn these into cheesy garlic breadsticks, we won't tell!

Olive oil, for oiling the pan

1 teaspoon instant yeast

2 tablespoons warm water

1 cup almond flour

1 teaspoon psyllium husk powder

1 teaspoon dried Italian herb seasoning

1 teaspoon garlic powder

1 teaspoon baking powder

1½ cups pre-shredded low-moisture part-skim mozzarella cheese

1 ounce cream cheese

1 large egg, beaten

1 tablespoon olive oil

1 tablespoon unsalted butter, melted

1 large clove garlic, peeled and crushed

½ teaspoon coarse salt

1 teaspoon minced fresh parsley

Per Serving
Calories: 206 | Fat: 16g |
Protein: 10g | Sodium: 347mg |
Fiber: 2g | Carbohydrates: 5g |
Net Carbohydrates: 3g | Sugar: 1g

1 Preheat oven to 400°F. Grease an 8" × 8" pan with oil.

2 To a small bowl, add yeast and warm water and stir to combine. Set aside until it's foamy, about 5–10 minutes.

3 In a medium bowl, whisk together almond flour, psyllium husk powder, Italian herb seasoning, garlic powder, and baking powder and set aside.

4 In a large microwave-safe bowl, add mozzarella and cream cheese. Microwave 60 seconds and then give it a stir, and continue microwaving in 20-second increments until cheese is fully melted and combined when stirred.

5 Stir yeast mixture into melted cheese until combined, and then stir in beaten egg until combined. Stir in almond flour mixture until it forms a dough.

6 Spread dough evenly into the greased pan. Make sure it is smooth and spread to the edges.

7 Pour oil over dough, spreading it out across entire dough.

8 Bake until dough is just starting to turn golden brown on top, about 12–15 minutes. Remove from oven.

9 In a small bowl, stir together melted butter and garlic. Drizzle garlic butter on top of dough. Sprinkle on coarse salt and parsley.

10 Return to oven and bake until the dough is golden on top and the garlic is fragrant, about 3–5 minutes.

11 Cut into eight sticks and serve warm.

Onion Rings

For those of you who used to order your burger with a side of onion rings before going keto, this recipe is for you. Crispy, crunchy, and delicious, these Onion Rings will satisfy your ASMR craving as well as your hankering for junk food!

Olive oil spray

1 cup almond flour

3 tablespoons grated Parmesan cheese

1 teaspoon garlic powder

¼ teaspoon ground black pepper

¹⁄₁₆ teaspoon cayenne pepper

2 large eggs

1 (10-ounce) yellow onion, peeled and sliced horizontally into ½"-thick circles

1 tablespoon coconut flour

1 Preheat oven to 425°F. Line a large baking sheet with parchment paper and spray it with olive oil.

2 In a shallow bowl, stir together almond flour, Parmesan, garlic powder, black pepper, and cayenne pepper.

3 In a separate shallow bowl, whisk together eggs.

4 Separate onion slices into rings. Pat them dry and add rings to a zip-top plastic bag along with coconut flour. Seal the bag and gently shake it to coat the rings.

5 Dip onion rings in egg, letting excess drip off, and then dip in almond flour mixture to coat. Arrange rings on the prepared baking sheet. Spray tops with olive oil.

6 Bake 10 minutes and then flip each onion ring over. Spray with olive oil again.

7 Return to oven and continue to bake until onion rings are golden on both sides, about 7–10 minutes more. Serve warm.

Per Serving
Calories: 117 | Fat: 8g | Protein: 5g | Sodium: 95mg | Fiber: 2g | Carbohydrates: 7g | Net Carbohydrates: 5g | Sugar: 2g

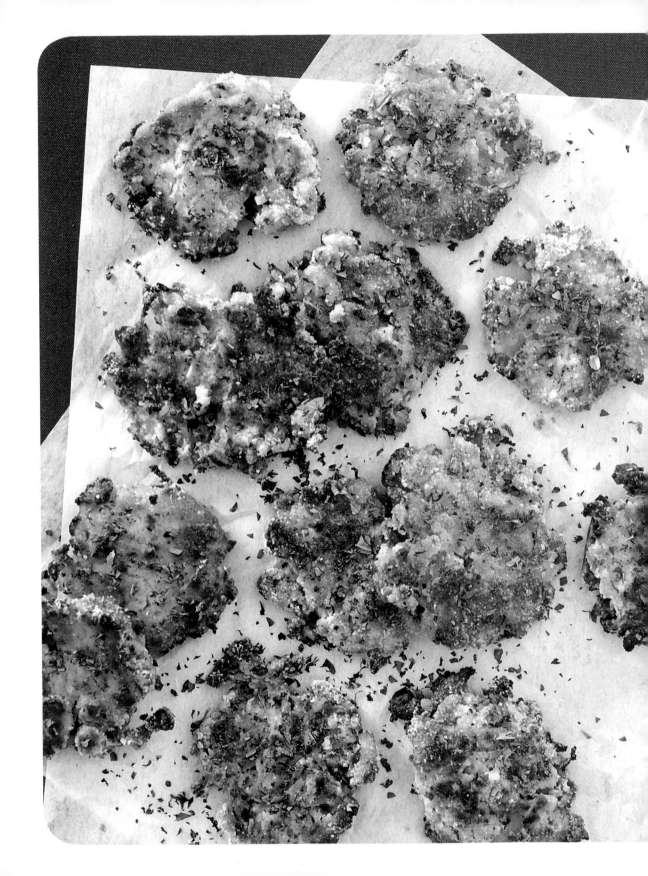

"Mac" and Cheese Bites

They might taste decadent, but our "Mac" and Cheese Bites also boast a healthy secret: cauliflower! The filling is rich, gooey, and ultra-cheesy, and the outside is crispy and golden. Serve them up with warmed no-sugar-added marinara sauce if you're into dipping.

COATING
½ cup almond flour
½ teaspoon garlic powder
½ teaspoon onion powder
½ teaspoon dried Italian herb seasoning
¼ teaspoon salt
¼ teaspoon ground black pepper

FILLING
3 cups cauliflower florets
1 large egg, lightly beaten
4 ounces shredded white Cheddar cheese
4½ tablespoons coconut flour
1 teaspoon onion powder
1 teaspoon garlic powder
⅛ teaspoon salt
⅛ teaspoon ground black pepper
1 cup pre-shredded low-moisture part-skim mozzarella cheese

OTHER
2 tablespoons extra-virgin olive oil, divided

1 *For the Coating:* In a shallow bowl, stir together all ingredients.

2 *For the Filling:* In a large microwave-safe bowl, place cauliflower and drape a paper towel over the top of the bowl. Microwave on high (don't add water) until the cauliflower is fork-tender but not mushy, about 5 minutes. Drain and cool slightly.

3 Mix egg into cauliflower, and then mix in Cheddar. Stir in coconut flour, onion powder, garlic powder, salt, and black pepper. Stir in mozzarella until well combined. It's okay if the cauliflower breaks up a bit. Refrigerate 10 minutes.

4 *To Bake:* Preheat oven to 425°F. Drizzle 1 tablespoon oil onto a large baking sheet and spread it around.

5 Scoop out 2 tablespoons of cauliflower mixture and roll it into a ball. Roll ball in Coating to lightly coat the outside. Place ball onto the prepared baking sheet and flatten it slightly to a patty. Repeat this process until all of cauliflower mixture is used, spacing cauliflower evenly apart on the sheet.

6 Bake until the patties are golden on the bottom, about 10–15 minutes. Remove sheet from oven and let it sit 2 minutes. Use a thin metal spatula to flip patties and drizzle remaining 1 tablespoon oil on top.

7 Return sheet to oven and bake until the patties are golden on the second side, about 8–10 minutes more. Serve warm.

Per Serving
Calories: 140 | Fat: 9g | Protein: 8g | Sodium: 227mg | Fiber: 2g | Carbohydrates: 6g | Net Carbohydrates: 4g | Sugar: 2g

Chicken Nugs

Let's just say chicken nugs from your favorite drive-through are a thing of the past! These oven-baked nugs are crunchy, flavorful, and extremely satisfying. To make them spicy nugs, add a bit more cayenne pepper and a dash of hot sauce in the egg mixture.

3 tablespoons olive oil, divided

½ cup almond flour

½ cup grated Parmesan cheese

½ tablespoon dried Italian herb seasoning

1 teaspoon onion powder

1 teaspoon garlic powder

½ teaspoon salt

½ teaspoon sweet paprika

¼ teaspoon ground black pepper

⅛ teaspoon cayenne pepper

2 large eggs

1 tablespoon water

1 pound boneless, skinless chicken breasts, cut into 2" × ½" pieces and patted dry

1 tablespoon coconut flour

1 Preheat oven to 400°F. Line a large baking sheet with foil, and brush the foil with 1 tablespoon oil.

2 In a shallow bowl, whisk together almond flour, Parmesan, Italian herb seasoning, onion powder, garlic powder, salt, paprika, black pepper, and cayenne pepper.

3 In a separate shallow bowl, crack eggs and lightly beat with water.

4 To a gallon-sized zip-top plastic bag, add chicken pieces and coconut flour and shake to coat chicken.

5 Shake off excess flour from a piece of chicken, dip it in egg, and then in almond flour mixture to coat, and place it on the prepared baking sheet. Continue until all the chicken pieces are breaded.

6 Drizzle remaining 2 tablespoons oil on top of breaded chicken.

7 Bake until the Chicken Nugs are golden on both sides, about 10 minutes, flipping once halfway through the cooking time. Serve warm.

Per Serving
Calories: 279 | Fat: 16g | Protein: 29g | Sodium: 452mg | Fiber: 2g | Carbohydrates: 4g | Net Carbohydrates: 2g | Sugar: 1g

Make Your Nugs a Meal!

You can easily make these Chicken Nugs a full meal by adding a green salad. Or to keep up the crunchy theme, roast broccoli or green beans in a 425°F oven to serve with the chicken (add a drizzle of olive oil and a sprinkle of salt and pepper; green beans roast about 15 minutes and broccoli florets roast about 25 minutes).

Garlic Parmesan Wings

These crispy fried wings with rich, buttery garlic flavor and nutty Parmesan cheese will have you licking your fingers to get every drop. You might only be able to find chicken wings that have the drumette and flat parts attached. If that's the case, just cut them apart before frying.

Oil, for frying

2 pounds chicken wings, a mix of drumettes and flats, patted dry and chilled

2 tablespoons salted butter

2 medium cloves garlic, peeled and crushed

4 tablespoons grated Parmesan cheese

2 teaspoons minced fresh parsley, for garnish

1 Add 3" oil to the bottom of a heavy-bottomed 5-quart pot. Heat oil over medium-high heat until it reaches 350°F. Carefully add half of chicken wings (straight from the refrigerator) and fry until golden, about 10 minutes. Place fried chicken wings on a paper towel-lined plate to drain excess oil. Fry remaining chicken wings the same way.

2 In a small skillet over medium heat, heat butter. Once melted, add garlic and cook 1 minute, stirring constantly. Remove from heat.

3 To a large bowl, add fried wings, garlic butter, and Parmesan and gently toss to coat wings.

4 Transfer wings to a serving platter and top with the parsley. Serve.

Per Serving
Calories: 471 | Fat: 39g | Protein: 28g | Sodium: 217mg | Fiber: 0g | Carbohydrates: 1g | Net Carbohydrates: 1g | Sugar: 0g

What Oil Should You Use?

For frying wings we recommend using an oil with a high smoke point, such as avocado oil or peanut oil.

Buffalo Wings

Buffalo Wings are an OG keto food from back in the day! It doesn't get much simpler: crispy skin outside, moist meat inside. You can adjust the amount of RedHot up if you want your wings spicier, or just add a touch of cayenne pepper when you're tossing the wings. Serve them with celery sticks and Blue Cheese (see recipe in this chapter) for the full effect.

Oil, for frying

2 pounds chicken wings, a mix of drumettes and flats, patted dry and chilled

2 tablespoons salted butter

2 tablespoons Frank's RedHot Original Cayenne Pepper Sauce

1 Add 3" oil to the bottom of a heavy-bottomed 5-quart pot. Heat oil over medium-high heat until it reaches 350°F. Carefully add half of chicken wings (straight from the refrigerator) and fry until golden, about 10 minutes. Place fried chicken wings on a paper towel–lined plate to drain excess oil. Fry remaining chicken wings the same way.

2 In a small skillet over medium heat, heat butter. Once melted, stir in hot sauce. Remove from heat.

3 To a large bowl, add fried wings and hot sauce mixture and gently toss to coat wings. Serve.

Per Serving
Calories: 456 | Fat: 38g | Protein: 27g | Sodium: 310mg | Fiber: 0g | Carbohydrates: 0g | Net Carbohydrates: 0g | Sugar: 0g

Like Your Wings Extra Crispy?

If you like your wings extra crispy, fry them for up to 15 minutes instead of 10!

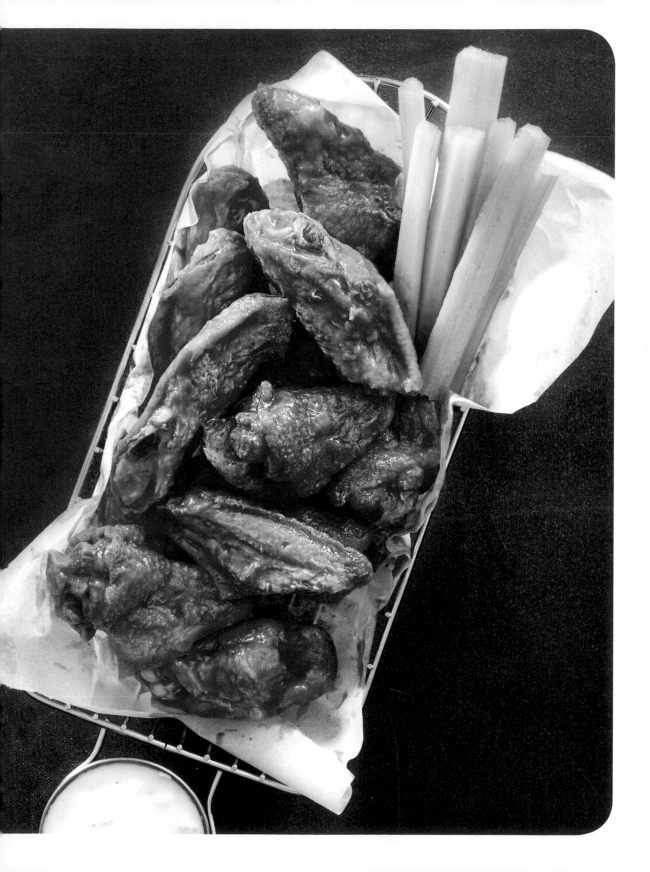

Sweet BBQ Wings

Savory Ranch (see recipe in this chapter) plus Sweet BBQ Wings are a match made in heaven! These wings are also a great pairing with our BBQ Chicken Pizza (see recipe in this chapter) for a homemade pizza and wing night.

Oil, for frying

2 pounds chicken wings, a mix of drumettes and flats, patted dry and chilled

⅓ cup Sweet BBQ Sauce (see recipe in this chapter)

1 Add 3" oil to the bottom of a heavy-bottomed 5-quart pot. Heat oil over medium-high heat until it reaches 350°F. Carefully add half of chicken wings (straight from the refrigerator) and fry until golden, about 10 minutes. Place fried chicken wings on a paper towel–lined plate to drain excess oil. Fry remaining chicken wings the same way.

2 To a large bowl, add fried wings and Sweet BBQ Sauce and gently toss to coat the wings. Serve.

Per Serving
Calories: 432 | Fat: 34g | Protein: 27g | Sodium: 208mg | Fiber: 0g | Carbohydrates: 9g | Net Carbohydrates: 2g | Sugar: 1g

Ranch

Creamy and velvety smooth, Ranch is just about everyone's favorite dressing! It goes way beyond salad, though. Ranch is great with Buffalo Wings or Chicken Nugs (see recipes in this chapter) for dipping, or with a Sub in a Tub (see Chapter 4) for drizzling on top. If you can't find fresh dill, you can use 1 teaspoon dried dill instead.

½ cup mayonnaise

¾ cup heavy whipping cream

2 tablespoons minced fresh parsley

2 teaspoons minced fresh dill

¾ teaspoon onion powder

¾ teaspoon garlic powder

¼ teaspoon salt

⅛ teaspoon ground black pepper

1 In a medium bowl, whisk together all ingredients.

2 Store in an airtight container in the refrigerator up to 1 week.

Per Serving
Calories: 137 | Fat: 14g | Protein: 1g | Sodium: 135mg | Fiber: 0g | Carbohydrates: 1g | Net Carbohydrates: 1g | Sugar: 1g

"Honey" Mustard

With three kinds of mustard, savory spices, and a touch of sweetness, this homemade low-carb "Honey" Mustard is every bit as delicious as its carb-laden counterpart! Use it to kick up a green salad, or serve it along with Onion Rings, "Mac" and Cheese Bites (see recipes in this chapter), or Club Sandwich Roll-Ups (see Chapter 4) for dunking.

¾ cup mayonnaise

3 tablespoons fresh lemon juice

½ tablespoon Dijon mustard

½ tablespoon stone-ground Dijon mustard

½ tablespoon yellow mustard

¼ teaspoon onion powder

¼ teaspoon garlic powder

¼ teaspoon sweet paprika

⅛ teaspoon salt

12 drops liquid stevia

1 In a medium bowl, whisk together all ingredients.

2 Store in an airtight container in the refrigerator up to 1 week.

Per Serving
Calories: 146 | Fat: 15g | Protein: 0g | Sodium: 224mg | Fiber: 0g | Carbohydrates: 1g | Net Carbohydrates: 1g | Sugar: 0g

**SERVES
6,
YIELDS
¾ CUP**

Sweet BBQ Sauce

If you're a fan of Sweet Baby Ray's, get ready to have your low-carb-loving mind blown! Sweet and tangy with a hint of spice and a touch of smoke, this Sweet BBQ Sauce recipe is our best replication of that classic favorite. You'll frequently find yourself making a batch to stash in the refrigerator because it's good on everything you can possibly put barbecue sauce on.

½ cup granulated (or crystalized) allulose sweetener

½ cup water

¼ cup tomato paste

¼ cup distilled vinegar

2 tablespoons apple cider vinegar

1 teaspoon liquid smoke

1 teaspoon molasses

1 teaspoon mustard powder

1 teaspoon garlic powder

¼ teaspoon smoked paprika

¼ teaspoon salt

⅛ teaspoon ground black pepper

⅛ teaspoon cayenne pepper

10 drops liquid stevia

1 To a medium saucepan over medium heat, add allulose and water. Bring to a full boil.

2 Whisk in all remaining ingredients, and bring back up to a full boil.

3 Let boil 3–5 minutes, whisking frequently, until it reaches your desired thickness.

4 Serve, or store covered in a glass container in the refrigerator up to 1 month.

Per Serving
Calories: 23 | Fat: 0g | Protein: 1g | Sodium: 184mg | Fiber: 1g | Carbohydrates: 20g | Net Carbohydrates: 3g | Sugar: 2g

Blue Cheese

Rich and flavorful, this Blue Cheese dressing is better than anything you can buy at the store. Use it instead of Ranch (see recipe in this chapter) for dipping chicken wings, or go Buffalo-style and serve Blue Cheese dressing along with pizza for dipping the crust.

⅓ cup mayonnaise

⅓ cup heavy whipping cream

⅓ cup blue cheese crumbles

2 teaspoons fresh lemon juice

1 teaspoon hot sauce

¼ teaspoon Worcestershire sauce

⅛ teaspoon onion powder

⅛ teaspoon garlic powder

⅛ teaspoon salt

⅛ teaspoon ground black pepper

1 In a medium bowl, whisk together all ingredients.

2 Store in an airtight container in the refrigerator up to 1 week.

Per Serving
Calories: 116 | Fat: 12g | Protein: 2g | Sodium: 183mg | Fiber: 0g | Carbohydrates: 1g | Net Carbohydrates: 1g | Sugar: 0g

CHAPTER 4

Burger Joints & Sub Shops

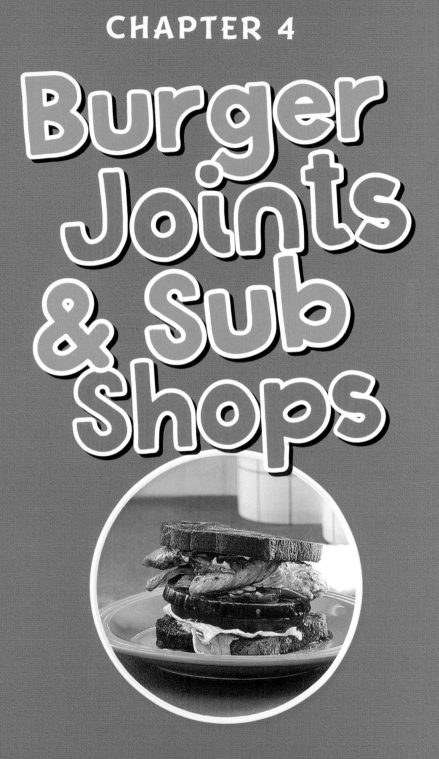

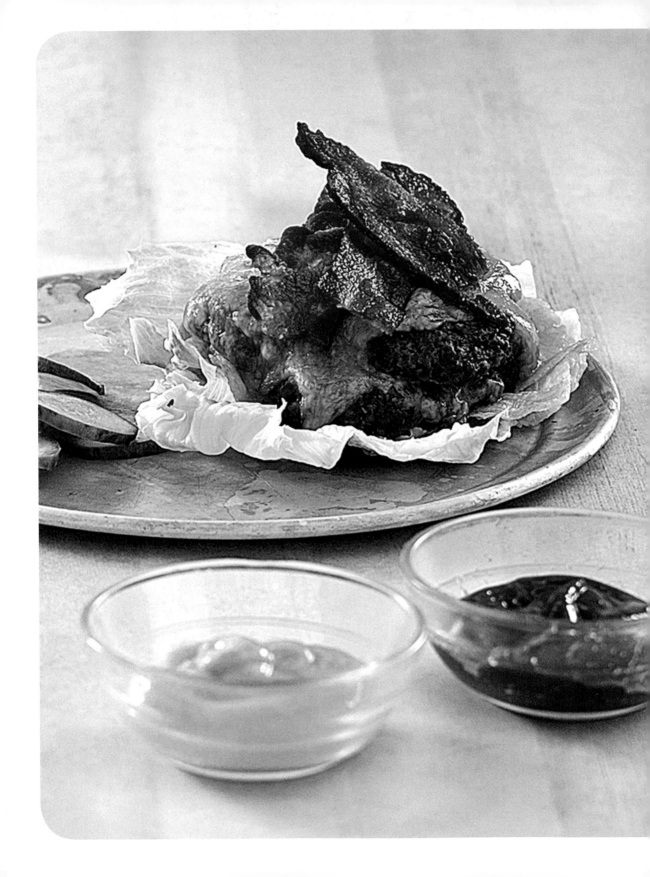

Bacon Double Cheeseburgers

Juicy and flavorful burgers are what we're going for here! And why have just a single burger when you can have a double?! Also, why have just a burger when you could make it a cheeseburger?!! And to really gild the lily, we added bacon. There's no way you're missing the carbs here.

1 pound 85% lean ground beef

1/2 small onion, peeled and grated

1 tablespoon Worcestershire sauce

1 1/2 teaspoons apple cider vinegar

1 teaspoon coconut aminos

1/4 teaspoon ground black pepper

1/8 teaspoon salt

1 tablespoon ghee, divided

4 (1-ounce) slices Cheddar cheese, cut in half

4 leaves iceberg lettuce

4 slices beef bacon, cooked until crispy

1 In a large bowl, add ground beef, onion, Worcestershire sauce, vinegar, coconut aminos, black pepper, and salt and use your hands to combine.

2 Divide meat into eight equal pieces, roll each into a ball, and flatten to a rectangle about 4 1/2" long × 3" wide.

3 In a cast iron skillet over medium-high heat, heat 1/2 tablespoon ghee. Once melted, add four patties and cook until browned on both sides, about 1–1 1/2 minutes per side, flipping once halfway through the cooking time. Top each with 1/2 slice cheese and transfer cooked patties to a plate.

4 Add remaining 1/2 tablespoon ghee and cook the remaining four patties the same way.

5 To serve, place each of the lettuce leaves on a plate. Top each with two cheeseburgers and a slice of bacon. Serve.

Per Serving
Calories: 457 | Fat: 31g | Protein: 34g | Sodium: 661mg | Fiber: 0g | Carbohydrates: 3g | Net Carbohydrates: 3g | Sugar: 1g

Southwestern Burgers

These perfectly spiced Southwestern Burgers are topped with a quick guacamole, sour cream, queso fresco, salsa, cilantro, and jalapeño for a fun Tex-Mex twist on burgers! They taste like tacos but in burger form, and are a great way to spice up both Taco Tuesday and burger night.

1 pound 85% lean ground beef

1 teaspoon onion powder

1 teaspoon garlic powder

1 teaspoon cumin

3/4 teaspoon plus 1/8 teaspoon salt, divided

1/2 teaspoon chili powder

1/4 teaspoon ground black pepper

1/2 tablespoon ghee

1 medium ripe Hass avocado, peeled and pitted

1 medium clove garlic, peeled and crushed

1 tablespoon fresh lemon juice

4 tablespoons full-fat sour cream

4 tablespoons crumbled queso fresco

4 tablespoons no-sugar-added salsa

2 tablespoons chopped fresh cilantro

1 medium jalapeño, thinly sliced

1 In a large bowl, add ground beef, onion powder, garlic powder, cumin, 3/4 teaspoon salt, chili powder, and black pepper and use your hands to combine.

2 Divide mixture into four equal pieces, roll each into a ball, and flatten into a patty.

3 In a cast iron skillet over medium-high heat, heat ghee. Once melted, add patties and cook until they're no longer pink in the center, about 4 minutes per side, flipping once halfway through the cooking time.

4 In a small bowl, mash avocado, garlic, lemon juice, and remaining 1/8 teaspoon salt together.

5 To serve, place each burger on a plate and top with 1/4 of mashed avocado mixture. Then top each with 1/4 of sour cream, queso fresco, salsa, cilantro, and jalapeño.

Per Serving
Calories: 336 | Fat: 20g | Protein: 25g | Sodium: 660mg | Fiber: 3g | Carbohydrates: 7g | Net Carbohydrates: 4g | Sugar: 1g

How to Make These Burgers a Full Meal

To make these a filling meal, we like to serve them on a bed of cauliflower rice with the toppings spilling over, almost like a burrito-in-a-bowl situation!

Smothered Burgers

The secret ingredient in this burger mixture is a splash of balsamic vinegar; it not only tenderizes the meat but also adds a hint of flavor and perfectly offsets the richness of the caramelized onions.

CARAMELIZED ONIONS

1 tablespoon olive oil

1/2 tablespoon unsalted butter

1 medium onion, peeled, quartered, and thinly sliced

1/4 teaspoon salt

1/8 teaspoon ground black pepper

BURGERS

1 pound 85% lean ground beef

1 tablespoon Worcestershire sauce

1 1/2 teaspoons balsamic vinegar

1 teaspoon coconut aminos

1/4 teaspoon ground black pepper

1/8 teaspoon salt

1 tablespoon ghee

2 tablespoons Sweet BBQ Sauce (see Chapter 3)

4 (1-ounce) slices pepper jack cheese

OTHER

4 Onion Rings (see Chapter 3)

1 *For the Caramelized Onions:* In a medium skillet over medium heat, heat oil and butter.

2 Add onion and cook until it's deep caramel in color, about 15–20 minutes, stirring occasionally. Add a splash of water or turn the heat down a little at any time if onions or the pan starts to get too dark.

3 Add salt and black pepper during the last 5 minutes of cooking, stirring occasionally.

4 *For the Burgers:* In a large bowl, add ground beef, Worcestershire sauce, vinegar, coconut aminos, black pepper, and salt and use your hands to combine.

5 Divide mixture into four equal pieces, roll each into a ball, and flatten into a patty.

6 In a cast iron skillet over medium-high heat, heat ghee. Once melted, add patties and cook until they're no longer pink in the center, about 4 minutes per side, flipping once halfway through the cooking time.

7 Remove skillet from heat, spread 1/2 tablespoon Sweet BBQ Sauce on top of each burger, and top each with 1 slice cheese. Drape a piece of foil on the top and let the cheese melt.

8 *To Serve:* Divide caramelized onions between the four burgers and place one Onion Ring on top of each. Serve.

Per Serving
Calories: 440 | Fat: 29g | Protein: 31g | Sodium: 605mg | Fiber: 1g | Carbohydrates: 11g | Net Carbohydrates: 6g | Sugar: 3g

Grilled Chicken Sammy

There's nothing earth-shattering about a chicken sandwich, but the simple flavors going on in this Grilled Chicken Sammy go together exceptionally well. Why reinvent the wheel when it comes to a classic that works, right?

1 pound chicken breast cutlets

½ teaspoon salt

¼ teaspoon ground black pepper

4 tablespoons mayonnaise

8 slices of your favorite keto bread, toasted

4 leaves iceberg lettuce

4 tomato slices

4 red onion slices

12 dill pickle chips

1 medium ripe Hass avocado, peeled, pitted, and thinly sliced

1 Season chicken with salt and black pepper. On a grill pan or outdoor grill over medium-high heat, grill chicken until it's fully cooked, about 2–4 minutes per side, flipping once halfway through the cooking time. There should be no pink in the center, and it should have an internal temperature of 165°F.

2 Spread ½ tablespoon mayonnaise on one side of each slice of bread. Top the mayonnaise side of each of 4 slices of bread with 1 lettuce leaf, 1 tomato slice, 1 onion slice, 3 pickle chips, ¼ of avocado slices, and ¼ of grilled chicken.

3 Place remaining bread slices on top of chicken, mayonnaise-side-down, to complete the sandwiches. Serve.

Per Serving
Calories: 404 | Fat: 26g | Protein: 37g | Sodium: 948mg | Fiber: 13g | Carbohydrates: 16g | Net Carbohydrates: 3g | Sugar: 2g

What Type of Keto Bread Should You Use?

With the increase in popularity of a ketogenic lifestyle, the sky is the limit in terms of bread options! You can find a variety of low-carb and keto breads (many of them with 0g net carbs) available at your regular grocery store or big-box store or online. Alternatively, if you have the time, you can bake a loaf of keto bread at home.

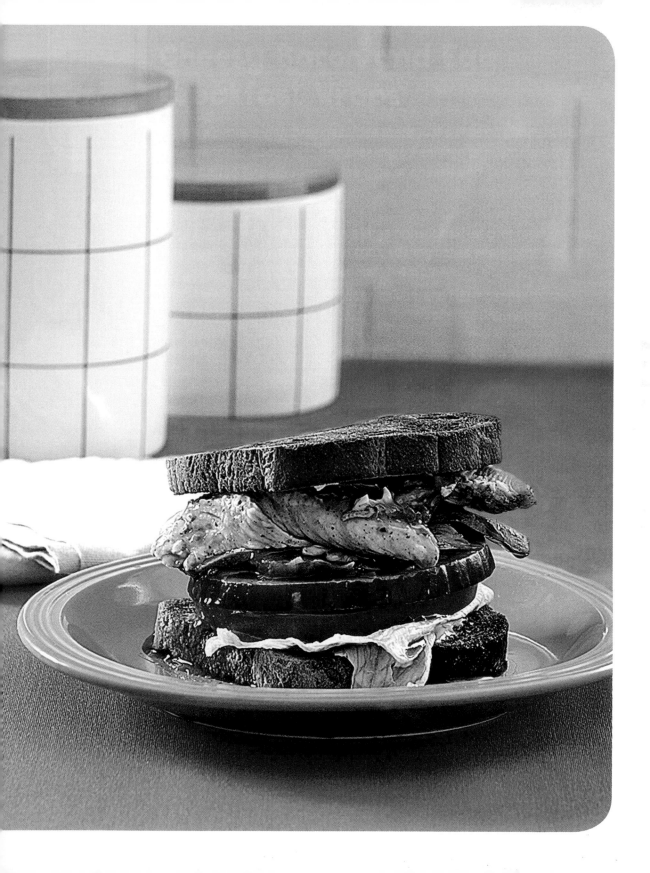

Sub in a Tub

Just like a lettuce-wrapped sandwich, a Sub in a Tub is a low-carb sub shop favorite! It has all your favorite sandwich fixings in a salad, and yes, go ahead and use your favorite kind of meat and cheese (note that the nutritional information may change if you do).

8 cups thinly sliced romaine lettuce

1 cup cherry tomatoes, halved

¼ cup thinly sliced red onion

4 dill pickle spears, chopped

8 ounces no-sugar-added deli-sliced turkey breast, chopped

4 ounces deli-sliced Swiss cheese, chopped

4 tablespoons Ranch (see Chapter 3)

1 Evenly divide lettuce between four bowls, and then divide tomatoes, onion, and pickle on top. Top with turkey and Swiss cheese.

2 Drizzle 1 tablespoon Ranch on top of each. Serve.

Per Serving
Calories: 258 | Fat: 15g | Protein: 21g | Sodium: 1,060mg | Fiber: 3g | Carbohydrates: 9g | Net Carbohydrates: 6g | Sugar: 4g

Oil on Your Subs?

We can help with that! Here's our favorite sub oil recipe: 3 tablespoons extra-virgin olive oil, 2 tablespoons white wine vinegar, 1 teaspoon crushed fresh garlic, 1 teaspoon dried Italian herb seasoning, and ¼ teaspoon salt. Whisk it all together and use it or store it up to 2 weeks in a covered jar in the refrigerator.

Fried Chicken Tenders Wrap

Crispy, crunchy chicken tenders are the star of the show in these delicious wraps! A few vegetables in the wraps also make it feel like you're getting in a balanced meal. Be sure to look for low-carb tortilla wraps that are 6"–8" in diameter so you can fold them over and eat them easier.

FRIED CHICKEN TENDERS

½ cup almond flour

½ cup grated Parmesan cheese

½ tablespoon dried Italian herb seasoning

1 teaspoon onion powder

1 teaspoon garlic powder

½ teaspoon salt

½ teaspoon sweet paprika

¼ teaspoon ground black pepper

⅛ teaspoon cayenne pepper

2 large eggs

1 tablespoon water

1 pound chicken tenders, patted dry

1 tablespoon coconut flour

Avocado oil, for frying

OTHER

4 (6"-8") low-carb tortilla wraps

4 teaspoons mayonnaise

1 cup baby spinach

¼ cup chopped tomato

¼ cup diced red onion

¼ cup shredded Cheddar cheese

1 *For the Fried Chicken Tenders:* In a shallow bowl, whisk together almond flour, Parmesan, Italian herb seasoning, onion powder, garlic powder, salt, paprika, black pepper, and cayenne pepper.

2 In a separate shallow bowl, crack eggs and lightly beat with the water.

3 To a gallon-sized zip-top plastic bag, add chicken pieces and coconut flour and shake to coat chicken.

4 Shake off excess coconut flour from a piece of chicken, dip it in egg and then in almond flour mixture to coat, and place it on a parchment paper–lined baking sheet. Continue until all the chicken pieces are breaded.

5 Add 2" oil to bottom of a heavy-bottomed 5-quart pot. Heat oil over medium-high heat until it reaches 365°F. Add ⅓ of chicken tenders and cook until golden on both sides, about 8–10 minutes, flipping once halfway through the cooking time. Place the fried chicken tenders on a paper towel–lined plate to drain excess oil. Fry remaining chicken tenders the same way, cooking ⅓ at a time.

6 *To Assemble the Wraps:* Lay one tortilla on a cutting board. Spread on 1 teaspoon mayonnaise. Top with ¼ cup spinach, 1 tablespoon tomato, 1 tablespoon onion, ¼ of fried chicken tenders, and 1 tablespoon Cheddar. Fold the wrap over onto itself to make a sandwich. Serve.

Per Serving
Calories: 496 | Fat: 37g | Protein: 27g | Sodium: 710mg | Fiber: 13g | Carbohydrates: 21g | Net Carbohydrates: 8g | Sugar: 2g

Club Sandwich Roll-Ups

Not only are these roll-ups a hit with adults, but they're also great finger food for toddlers! They work well for a quick meal like lunch at the office or as a snack when you're watching TV. And they're perfect for meal prep; you can make them up to 3 days in advance and stash them in the refrigerator!

8 ounces no-sugar-added deli-sliced turkey breast

2 tablespoons mayonnaise

4 (1-ounce) slices Cheddar cheese

8 slices beef bacon, cooked until crispy

1 cup thinly sliced iceberg lettuce

1/4 cup chopped tomato

1/4 cup diced red onion

1 Divide turkey into four 2-ounce portions. Spread out each 2-ounce portion of turkey and lay it flat on a cutting board.

2 Spread 1/2 tablespoon mayonnaise on top of each turkey portion.

3 Place 1 slice cheese and 2 slices bacon on top of each.

4 Sprinkle 1/4 cup lettuce, 1 tablespoon tomato, and 1 tablespoon onion on each.

5 Roll up the turkey so the fillings are inside. Serve.

Per Serving
Calories: 422 | Fat: 32g | Protein: 27g | Sodium: 1,439mg | Fiber: 0g | Carbohydrates: 3g | Net Carbohydrates: 3g | Sugar: 1g

Thick or Thin Deli Turkey?

When you're making roll-ups out of deli meat, we recommend having the meat sliced to a medium thickness. Having the meat cut very thin or shaved will make it very hard to roll them up!

Pork Rind "Poutine"

Have you tried the Canadian classic poutine? It's a dish of French fries, brown gravy, and cheese curds that originated in Quebec. It's an easy recipe to keto-fy using pork rinds in place of French fries! We use beef gelatin to make the gravy, and it thickens more as it cools. If it gets cold it will gel and need to be reheated.

GRAVY

6 tablespoons cold water

1 tablespoon beef gelatin

½ tablespoon ghee

1 cup beef stock

½ teaspoon Worcestershire sauce

⅛ teaspoon onion powder

⅛ teaspoon garlic powder

1/16 teaspoon ground black pepper

OTHER

4 ounces unflavored pork rinds

8 ounces Cheddar cheese curds

1 tablespoon minced chives

1 *For the Gravy:* In a small bowl, add cold water. Sprinkle gelatin on top and stir to combine. Let it sit 5 minutes to bloom the gelatin.

2 To a medium saucepan over medium-high heat, add ghee, beef stock, Worcestershire sauce, onion powder, garlic powder, and black pepper.

3 Bring to a boil, add bloomed gelatin, and then let it boil 5–10 minutes, until it's reduced to about ¾ cup.

4 Remove from heat and cool about 10 minutes. It will thicken as it cools.

5 *To Serve:* Preheat oven to 425°F. Spread out pork rinds in a 9" × 13" casserole dish. Bake 5 minutes.

6 Remove from oven, drizzle on gravy, and sprinkle on cheese curds. Return to oven for 2 minutes.

7 Remove from oven and sprinkle on chives. Serve.

Per Serving
Calories: 206 | Fat: 14g | Protein: 16g | Sodium: 509mg | Fiber: 0g | Carbohydrates: 2g | Net Carbohydrates: 2g | Sugar: 0g

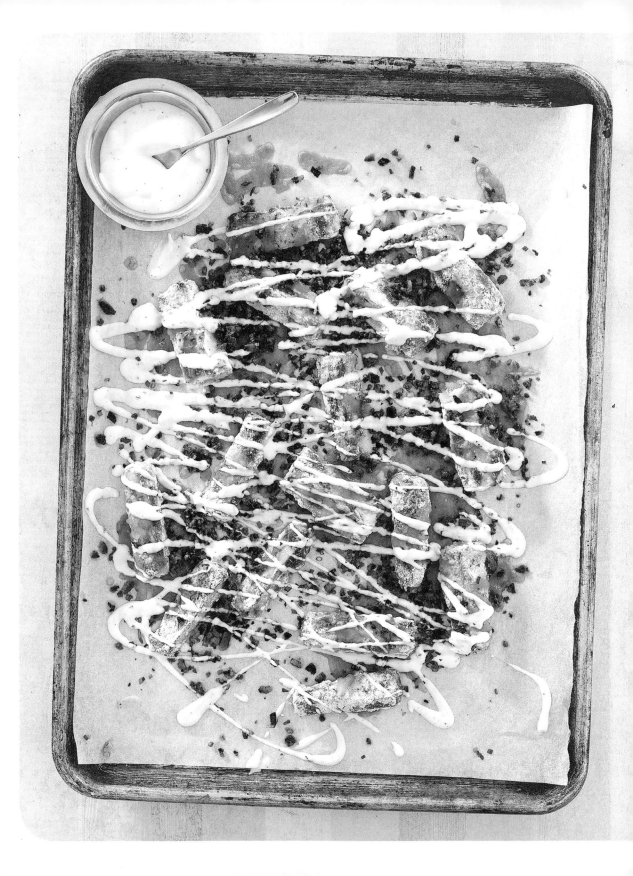

Loaded Zucchini Fries

Crispy and golden, these flavorful Loaded Zucchini Fries are a surprise for two reasons. First, you'd never guess that they're baked and not deep-fried with their perfectly crunchy exterior. And second, the fact that they're keto and gluten-free will blow your mind!

ZUCCHINI FRIES

Avocado oil spray

1½ ounces pork rinds

2 tablespoons grated Parmesan cheese

¾ cup almond flour

1 teaspoon dried Italian herb seasoning

1 teaspoon garlic powder

2 large eggs

1 pound zucchini (about 3 smallish zucchini)

2 teaspoons coconut flour

OTHER

4 ounces shredded Cheddar cheese

4 slices beef bacon, cooked until crispy, and then crumbled

2 tablespoons minced fresh chives, for garnish

2 tablespoons Ranch, for drizzling on top (see Chapter 3)

Per Serving
Calories: 225 | Fat: 17g |
Protein: 12g | Sodium: 359mg |
Fiber: 2g | Carbohydrates: 4g |
Net Carbohydrates: 2g | Sugar: 2g

1 *For the Zucchini Fries:* Preheat oven to 425°F. Line a large baking sheet with parchment paper or foil and lightly spray it with avocado oil.

2 Process pork rinds in a food processor until they form crumbs. Add Parmesan, almond flour, Italian herb seasoning, and garlic powder and pulse a couple times to combine. Transfer to a shallow bowl and set aside.

3 Beat eggs in a separate shallow bowl and set aside.

4 Trim both ends off zucchini. Cut zucchini in half across the middle, and then cut each half into quarters lengthwise, so you end up with four "logs." Pat zucchini dry with paper towels.

5 Add zucchini to a large zip-top plastic bag. Sprinkle in coconut flour, seal the bag, and toss to coat zucchini.

6 Working with one zucchini log at a time, shake off excess coconut flour, dip it in egg (and let excess egg drip off), and then coat it in pork rind mixture. Place it on the prepared baking sheet. Continue this way until all zucchini is coated.

7 Lightly spray the tops of zucchini fries with avocado oil.

8 Bake until zucchini is golden and crispy, about 25 minutes, flipping once halfway through the cooking time.

9 *To Load the Fries:* Once zucchini fries are cooked, use a metal spatula to push them to the center of the baking sheet. Sprinkle on Cheddar and bacon.

10 Broil until cheese is melted, about 2–3 minutes.

11 Sprinkle chives on top and drizzle with Ranch. Serve warm.

Bacon-Wrapped Jalapeño Poppers

These Bacon-Wrapped Jalapeño Poppers are smoky, cheesy, and a little spicy! Two types of cheese, bacon, and jalapeño peppers are all you need for one of the best (and easiest) appetizers. Serve these up with Buffalo Wings (see Chapter 3) for an easy pizzeria-style meal at home, or include them as part of a football game night spread.

8 large jalapeño peppers (each about 4" long)

3 ounces shredded sharp yellow Cheddar cheese

3 ounces full-fat cream cheese

½ teaspoon garlic powder

8 slices beef bacon

Avocado oil spray

1 Preheat oven to 400°F.

2 Cut a thin slit down the length of each pepper and carefully remove the inner ribs and seeds, trying to keep the pepper itself as intact as possible.

3 In a small bowl, use a fork to mash together Cheddar, cream cheese, and garlic powder.

4 Stuff cheese mixture into each pepper, closing up each pepper as much as you can.

5 Wrap a slice of raw bacon around the outside of each pepper, securing with a toothpick if necessary.

6 Lightly spray each popper with avocado oil.

7 Arrange poppers on a large baking sheet and bake until the bacon is crispy, about 20 minutes. You can broil poppers for a couple minutes at the end if you want to brown them more. Serve warm.

Per Serving
Calories: 184 | Fat: 15g | Protein: 8g | Sodium: 372mg | Fiber: 0g | Carbohydrates: 2g | Net Carbohydrates: 2g | Sugar: 1g

Can't Find Large Jalapeño Peppers?

The size of jalapeños can vary greatly. If you can't find large jalapeños, you can use 16 small ones (for 2 poppers per serving), each wrapped with half a slice of bacon. Start checking them to see if they're done after 15 minutes.

CHAPTER 5
Asian Takeout

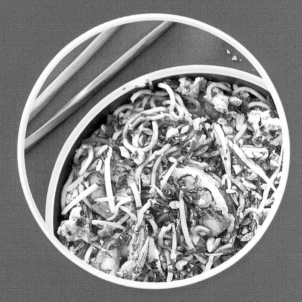

Fried "Rice"

When it comes to takeout night, Chinese food is always a favorite. Try this Fried "Rice" and it will become your go-to instead of reaching for the takeout menu. We recommend frying the eggs "over easy" so you can enjoy runny yolk dripping down into the cauliflower rice. To add more protein, add cooked, chopped chicken or steak at the same time you add the riced cauliflower; just note that this will change the nutritional information.

2 tablespoons unsalted butter

1 tablespoon avocado oil

5 ounces shitake mushrooms, thinly sliced

1/2 medium yellow onion, peeled and chopped small

2 large stalks celery, thinly sliced

3 large cloves garlic, peeled and minced

1 tablespoon grated fresh ginger

2 1/2 cups riced cauliflower

3 tablespoons tamari sauce

1/2 teaspoon salt

1/4 teaspoon ground black pepper

2 medium scallions, green and white parts, thinly sliced

1/2 tablespoon toasted sesame oil, for garnish

5 large eggs, fried in 1 tablespoon avocado oil

1 To a large skillet over medium to medium-high heat, add butter and avocado oil. Once butter is melted, add mushrooms and onion and cook until softened but not browned, about 6–8 minutes, stirring occasionally.

2 Stir in celery, garlic, and ginger and cook 2 minutes, stirring constantly.

3 Add cauliflower, turn the heat up to high, and cook 1–2 minutes, stirring constantly.

4 Stir in tamari sauce, salt, and black pepper and turn off heat.

5 Sprinkle on scallions and drizzle on sesame oil. Serve warm, topped with 1 fried egg per serving.

Per Serving
Calories: 205 | Fat: 15g | Protein: 10g | Sodium: 958mg | Fiber: 2g | Carbohydrates: 8g | Net Carbohydrates: 6g | Sugar: 3g

Make It Spicy Without Adding Carbs

A lot of store-bought hot sauces are low in carbohydrates; just be sure to read the labels to see what fits into your macros. One of our favorites is sambal oelek (also called chili garlic sauce), which has 0g net carbs per 1-teaspoon serving.

General Tso's Chicken

It's crispy, it's spicy, it's savory, it goes really well with our Fried "Rice" in this chapter…it's General Tso's Chicken! The trick to getting this chicken just right is to shallow-fry it. We tried cooking it in the oven, and it just doesn't do the recipe justice.

CRISPY CHICKEN

½ cup almond flour

4 tablespoons coconut flour

½ teaspoon salt

½ teaspoon ground black pepper

1½ pounds boneless, skinless chicken thighs, cut into 1" pieces

Avocado oil, for shallow frying

GENERAL TSO'S SAUCE

1 tablespoon avocado oil

3 medium cloves garlic, peeled and crushed

1 tablespoon grated fresh ginger

3 tablespoons tamari sauce

2 tablespoons rice vinegar

2 tablespoons chili garlic sauce

2 tablespoons granulated (or crystalized) allulose sweetener

1 teaspoon toasted sesame oil

½ teaspoon crushed red pepper flakes

2 medium scallions, green and white parts, thinly sliced

1 *For the Crispy Chicken:* In a shallow bowl, stir together almond flour, coconut flour, salt, and black pepper.

2 Pat chicken dry with a couple paper towels. Roll chicken in almond flour mixture to lightly coat all the pieces.

3 To a large, heavy-bottomed skillet, add enough avocado oil to coat the bottom evenly. Heat oil over medium to medium-high heat.

4 Once hot, add chicken in a single layer, being careful not to overcrowd the pan. Cook until golden outside and no longer pink in the center, about 10–12 minutes, flipping once halfway through the cooking time. Adjust heat down as necessary if chicken starts to cook too fast.

5 Once cooked, transfer chicken to a paper towel–lined plate to drain excess oil, and drape the top with a piece of foil to help keep it warm. Cook remaining chicken the same way, adding more oil if needed.

6 *For the General Tso's Sauce:* To a small skillet over medium heat, add avocado oil. Once hot, add garlic and ginger and cook 30 seconds, stirring constantly. Whisk in tamari sauce, vinegar, chili garlic sauce, allulose, sesame oil, and red pepper flakes. Bring to a boil, and then remove from heat. Stir in scallions.

7 *To Serve:* Transfer chicken to a serving plate and drizzle General Tso's Sauce on top. Serve immediately.

Per Serving

Calories: 322 | Fat: 21g | Protein: 25g | Sodium: 921mg | Fiber: 2g | Carbohydrates: 8g | Net Carbohydrates: 2g | Sugar: 1g

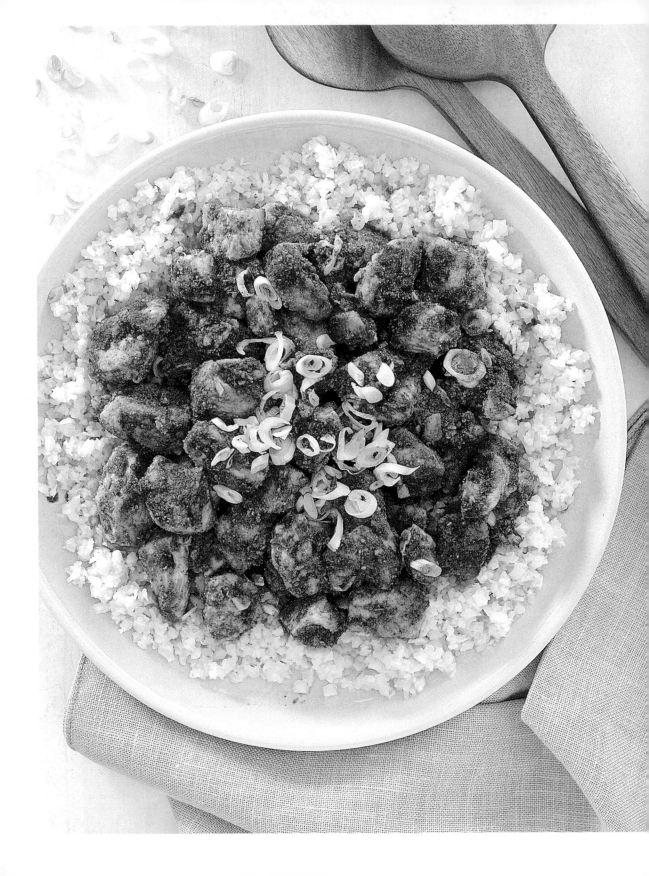

Orange Chicken

We know what you're wondering…how on earth did they keto-fy Orange Chicken?! This savory dish is usually on the sweeter side with a touch of spice. Instead of using whole oranges or orange juice, we use orange zest for a pop of zingy flavor with many fewer carbs!

CRISPY CHICKEN

½ cup almond flour

4 tablespoons coconut flour

½ teaspoon salt

½ teaspoon ground black pepper

1½ pounds boneless, skinless chicken thighs, cut into 1" pieces

Avocado oil, for shallow frying

ORANGE SAUCE

1 tablespoon avocado oil

3 medium cloves garlic, peeled and crushed

1 tablespoon grated fresh ginger

3 tablespoons tamari sauce

2 tablespoons rice vinegar

1 tablespoon sriracha

2 tablespoons granulated (or crystalized) allulose sweetener

1 teaspoon toasted sesame oil

1½ tablespoons grated fresh orange zest

2 medium scallions, green and white parts, thinly sliced

1 *For the Crispy Chicken:* In a shallow bowl, stir together almond flour, coconut flour, salt, and black pepper.

2 Pat chicken dry with paper towels. Roll chicken in almond flour mixture to lightly coat all the pieces.

3 In a large, heavy-bottomed skillet, add enough avocado oil to coat the bottom evenly. Heat oil over medium to medium-high heat.

4 Once hot, add chicken in a single layer, being careful not to overcrowd the pan. Cook until golden outside and no longer pink in the center, about 10–12 minutes, flipping once halfway through the cooking time. Adjust heat down as necessary if chicken starts to cook too fast.

5 Once cooked, transfer chicken to a paper towel–lined plate to drain excess oil, and drape the top with a piece of foil to help keep it warm. Cook remaining chicken the same way, adding more oil if needed.

6 *For the Orange Sauce:* In a small skillet over medium heat, add avocado oil. Once hot, add garlic and ginger and cook 30 seconds, stirring constantly. Whisk in tamari sauce, vinegar, sriracha, allulose, and sesame oil. Bring to a boil, and then remove from heat. Stir in orange zest and scallions.

7 *To Serve:* Transfer chicken to a serving plate and drizzle Orange Sauce on top. Serve immediately.

Per Serving

Calories: 326 | Fat: 21g | Protein: 25g | Sodium: 856mg | Fiber: 2g | Carbohydrates: 9g | Net Carbohydrates: 3g | Sugar: 1g

Sesame Chicken

Who says kids don't like keto-friendly foods? Make this dish for your kiddos and watch them eat it all and ask for seconds. With crispy chicken and a sweet and savory sesame sauce, this is a meal everyone will want in your regular dinner rotation.

CRISPY CHICKEN

½ cup almond flour

4 tablespoons coconut flour

½ teaspoon salt

½ teaspoon ground black pepper

1½ pounds boneless, skinless chicken thighs, cut into 1" pieces

Avocado oil, for shallow frying

SESAME SAUCE

1 tablespoon avocado oil

3 medium cloves garlic, peeled and crushed

3 tablespoons sugar-free ketchup

3 tablespoons tamari sauce

2 tablespoons rice vinegar

2 tablespoons keto brown sugar

½ tablespoon toasted sesame oil

1 tablespoon sesame seeds

2 medium scallions, green and white parts, thinly sliced

1 *For the Crispy Chicken:* In a shallow bowl, stir together almond flour, coconut flour, salt, and black pepper.

2 Pat chicken dry with a couple paper towels.

3 Roll chicken in almond flour mixture to lightly coat all the pieces.

4 In a large, heavy-bottomed skillet, add enough avocado oil to coat the bottom evenly. Heat oil over medium to medium-high heat.

5 Once hot, add chicken in a single layer, being careful not to overcrowd the pan. Cook until golden outside and no longer pink in the center, about 10–12 minutes, flipping once halfway through the cooking time. Adjust the heat down as necessary if chicken starts to cook too fast.

6 Once cooked, transfer chicken to a paper towel–lined plate to drain excess oil, and drape the top with a piece of foil to help keep it warm. Cook remaining chicken the same way, adding more oil if needed.

7 *For the Sesame Sauce:* To a small skillet over medium heat, add avocado oil. Once hot, add garlic and cook 30 seconds, stirring constantly. Whisk in ketchup, tamari sauce, vinegar, brown sugar, sesame oil, and sesame seeds. Bring to a boil, and then remove from heat. Stir in the scallions.

8 *To Serve:* Transfer chicken to a serving plate and drizzle Sesame Sauce on top. Serve immediately.

Per Serving
Calories: 334 | Fat: 22g | Protein: 25g | Sodium: 804mg | Fiber: 2g | Carbohydrates: 9g | Net Carbohydrates: 3g | Sugar: 1g

Singapore Noodles

Curry gives this classic noodle dish its golden hue, complex aroma, and distinctive flavor. Curry is a strong flavor and can be overpowering if you're not careful, so we like to start with a small amount and add more to taste.

2 tablespoons avocado oil, divided

2 large eggs, lightly beaten

6 ounces small raw shrimp, peeled and deveined

1/2 small yellow onion, peeled and thinly sliced

1/4 cup thinly sliced red bell pepper

1/4 cup thinly sliced green bell pepper

3 cups thinly sliced Napa cabbage

3 medium cloves garlic, peeled and crushed

1 teaspoon grated fresh ginger

2 tablespoons tamari sauce

1 tablespoon rice vinegar

1 1/2 teaspoons keto brown sugar, lightly packed

1/2 teaspoon curry powder

1/4 teaspoon crushed red pepper flakes

1/8 teaspoon ground white pepper

1 (400-gram) can Palmini hearts of palm linguine, rinsed and drained

1 tablespoon toasted sesame oil

1 medium scallion, thinly sliced

1 Heat a large nonstick skillet over high heat. Once the pan is very hot, add 1/2 tablespoon avocado oil and turn the heat down to medium-high. Add eggs and scramble to break them up. Let cook until they are set, about 1 minute. Transfer eggs to a small bowl and set aside.

2 To same skillet, add 1 tablespoon avocado oil. Once hot, add shrimp and cook until it turns pink, about 2–3 minutes, stirring occasionally. Transfer shrimp to a medium bowl and set aside.

3 To same skillet, add remaining 1/2 tablespoon avocado oil, onion, red bell pepper, green bell pepper, and cabbage. Turn heat down to medium. Cook until vegetables are just starting to soften, about 1–2 minutes, stirring frequently.

4 Stir in garlic, ginger, tamari sauce, vinegar, brown sugar, curry powder, red pepper flakes, and white pepper, and cook 30 seconds, stirring constantly.

5 Add Palmini linguine and cook 2 minutes, stirring frequently. Stir in scrambled eggs and cooked shrimp. Remove from heat.

6 Top with sesame oil and scallion. Serve.

Per Serving
Calories: 273 | Fat: 17g | Protein: 16g | Sodium: 1,052mg | Fiber: 5g | Carbohydrates: 16g | Net Carbohydrates: 9g | Sugar: 4g

Spring Roll in a Bowl

Loosely inspired by Vietnamese noodle salad, this dish is an herbaceous combination of vegetables that packs a ton of flavor and crunch! If you want "noodles" in your bowl, you can spiralize daikon radish or zucchini. And to bump up the protein, feel free to add whatever your favorite protein is (a couple of our favorite proteins for this are grilled chicken thighs and slow-cooked beef short ribs).

SAUCE

2 tablespoons avocado oil

2 tablespoons fresh lime juice

1½ tablespoons tamari sauce

1 tablespoon rice vinegar

1 tablespoon keto brown sugar

1 medium clove garlic, peeled and crushed

1 teaspoon grated fresh ginger

1 teaspoon toasted sesame oil

½ teaspoon white sesame seeds

½ teaspoon black sesame seeds

⅛ teaspoon crushed red pepper flakes

1/16 teaspoon ground white pepper

SALAD

3 cups thinly sliced Napa cabbage

1 cup thinly sliced cucumber

1 cup bean sprouts

¼ cup julienned carrot

1 medium ripe Hass avocado, halved, pitted, and thinly sliced

¼ cup whole fresh mint leaves

¼ cup whole fresh cilantro leaves

¼ cup whole fresh Thai basil leaves

1 medium scallion, green and white parts, thinly sliced

1 *For the Sauce:* In a small bowl, whisk together all ingredients and set aside.

2 *For the Salad:* Divide cabbage between two shallow bowls and top each with half of cucumber, bean sprouts, carrot, avocado, mint, cilantro, basil, and scallion. Serve or cover each salad and store in the refrigerator up to 2 hours before serving.

3 *To Serve:* Drizzle half the sauce on top of each salad and serve immediately.

Per Serving
Calories: 332 | Fat: 26g | Protein: 6g | Sodium: 878mg | Fiber: 9g | Carbohydrates: 27g | Net Carbohydrates: 12g | Sugar: 7g

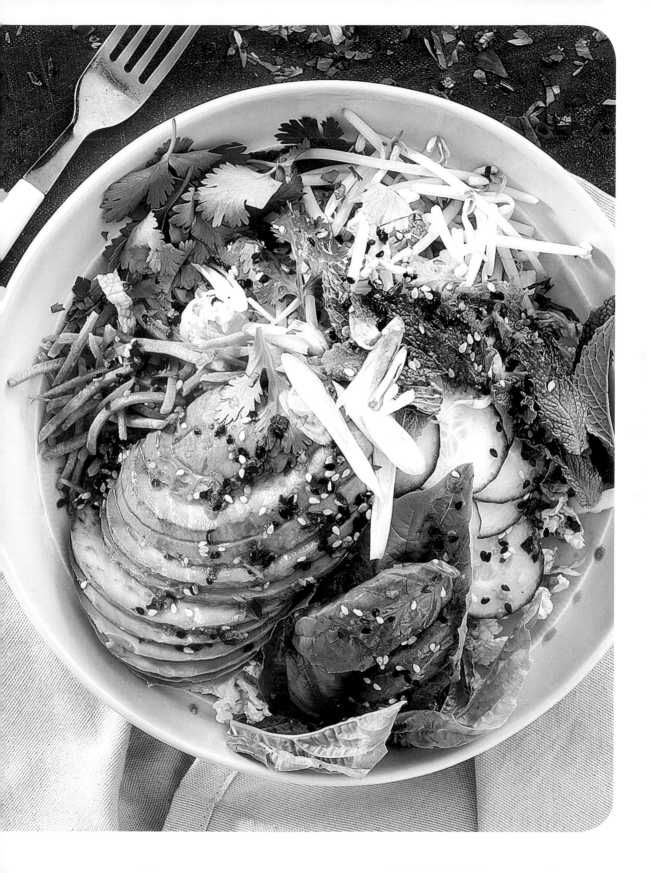

Egg Roll in a Bowl

An Egg Roll in a Bowl is basically stir-fry that's flavored the same way as egg roll filling. It keeps well in the refrigerator up to 4 days and is a good one to meal prep for lunches on busy days.

1½ pounds 85% lean ground beef

2 pounds green cabbage, thinly sliced (about ½ a medium head)

1 small yellow onion, peeled and thinly sliced

1 medium carrot, peeled and thinly sliced

5 large cloves garlic, peeled and minced

1 tablespoon grated fresh ginger

2 tablespoons tamari sauce

2 tablespoons rice vinegar

2 tablespoons keto brown sugar

1 tablespoon chili garlic sauce

4 teaspoons sesame seeds, divided

½ teaspoon salt

¼ teaspoon ground black pepper

1 teaspoon toasted sesame oil

1 medium scallion, green and white parts, thinly sliced

1 Heat a large, deep skillet over medium-high heat. Once hot, add ground beef and cook until browned, about 8 minutes, stirring occasionally.

2 Add cabbage, onion, and carrot and cook until vegetables are softened and starting to caramelize in spots, about 5 minutes, stirring occasionally. Add garlic and ginger and cook 1 minute more, stirring constantly.

3 Turn off heat and stir in tamari sauce, vinegar, brown sugar, chili garlic sauce, 3 teaspoons sesame seeds, salt, and black pepper.

4 Transfer to a serving dish and top with remaining 1 teaspoon sesame seeds, sesame oil, and scallion. Serve.

Per Serving
Calories: 267 | Fat: 11g | Protein: 24g | Sodium: 688mg | Fiber: 5g | Carbohydrates: 17g | Net Carbohydrates: 8g | Sugar: 6g

Keto Lo Mein

Is it really Chinese takeout night if there isn't lo mein?! This keto version comes together in just 20 minutes so you can recreate your takeout favorite in less time than it would take to order it and have dinner delivered! To bump up the protein and make it a more satisfying meal, we like to sauté ¾ pound of boneless, skinless chicken thighs to serve with this dish.

1½ tablespoons olive oil

½ small yellow onion, peeled and thinly sliced

¼ cup thinly sliced red bell pepper

¼ cup thinly sliced green bell pepper

1 cup snow peas

3 medium cloves garlic, peeled and crushed

1 teaspoon grated fresh ginger

2 tablespoons tamari sauce

1 tablespoon rice vinegar

1½ teaspoons keto brown sugar, lightly packed

⅛ teaspoon ground white pepper

1 (400-gram) can Palmini hearts of palm linguine, rinsed and drained

1 tablespoon toasted sesame oil

1 medium scallion, thinly sliced

½ teaspoon sesame seeds

1 Heat a medium to large skillet over high heat. Once the pan is very hot, add olive oil and turn heat down to medium. Add onion, red bell pepper, green bell pepper, and snow peas. Cook until vegetables are just starting to soften, about 1–2 minutes, stirring frequently.

2 Stir in garlic, ginger, tamari sauce, vinegar, brown sugar, and white pepper and cook 30 seconds, stirring constantly.

3 Add Palmini linguine and cook 2 minutes, stirring frequently. Remove from heat.

4 Top with sesame oil, scallion, and sesame seeds. Serve.

Per Serving
Calories: 140 | Fat: 11g | Protein: 3g | Sodium: 672mg | Fiber: 2g | Carbohydrates: 9g | Net Carbohydrates: 5g | Sugar: 2g

What Is Palmini?!

Palmini linguine is a keto "pasta" made out of hearts of palm! It comes in a can or in a pouch, and you can usually find it in the canned vegetable aisle of your regular grocery store. It also comes in other shapes, such as lasagna and angel hair. What we love about it is that it looks very similar to regular pasta, doesn't have a strong flavor of its own, cooks up quick, and has just 2g net carbs per serving!

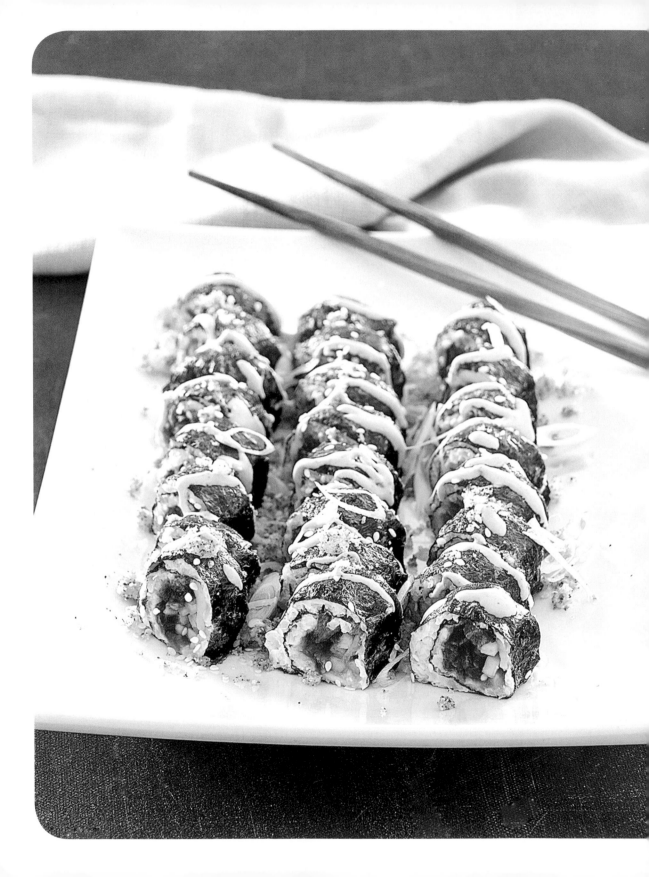

Crazy "Sushi" Roll

SERVES 4

Yes, you can have sushi with rice, sauce, and crunchy topping! Of course, they're all keto-fied. Cauliflower rice, an easy spicy mayonnaise, and our personal favorite, crispy fried onions stand in for crispy tempura topping. Sushi lover satisfaction is guaranteed. You can find most of these ingredients in the international aisle at a regular grocery store, in an Asian supermarket, or online.

CAULIFLOWER RICE

2 teaspoons avocado oil

2 cups riced cauliflower

3 ounces cream cheese

CRUNCHY ONION TOPPING

3 tablespoons minced white onion

¼ teaspoon coconut flour

⅛ teaspoon salt

2 tablespoons avocado oil

SPICY MAYONNAISE

⅓ cup mayonnaise

¾ teaspoon chili garlic sauce

¾ teaspoon rice vinegar

¾ teaspoon tamari sauce

½ teaspoon toasted sesame oil

¼ teaspoon powdered allulose sweetener

1/16 teaspoon ground white pepper

SPICY TUNA

8 ounces sashimi-grade tuna, chopped into ⅛" pieces

3 tablespoons chili garlic sauce

Ingredients continued on the next page ▶

1 *For the Cauliflower Rice:* Heat a large skillet over medium heat. Add avocado oil and, once hot, add cauliflower. Cook until cauliflower is starting to soften but not brown, about 3–5 minutes, stirring frequently.

2 Remove from heat and stir in cream cheese until well mixed. Cool to room temperature and then refrigerate 15 minutes to chill.

3 *For the Crunchy Onion Topping:* In a small bowl, toss together onion, coconut flour, and salt to coat the onion.

4 In a small skillet over medium heat, heat avocado oil. Once hot, add onion mixture. Cook until onion is crispy, about 3–4 minutes, stirring constantly.

5 Pour onions onto a paper towel–lined plate to drain excess oil. Cool to room temperature.

6 *For the Spicy Mayonnaise:* In a small bowl, whisk together all ingredients. Cover and refrigerate until ready to serve.

7 *For the Spicy Tuna:* In a medium bowl, add all ingredients and gently stir until well combined. Cover and refrigerate until ready to serve.

8 *To Assemble the Sushi Rolls:* Lay nori sheets on a cutting board or countertop. Divide cauliflower rice mixture evenly between sheets and spread it out evenly on each.

Continued on the next page ▶

1 tablespoon tamari sauce

½ tablespoon toasted sesame oil

1 medium scallion, green and white parts, thinly sliced

1 teaspoon sesame seeds

OTHER

4 (7" × 8") sheets nori

¼ medium English cucumber, julienned

1 medium ripe Hass avocado, peeled, pitted, and very thinly sliced

1 medium scallion, green and white parts, thinly sliced

1 teaspoon sesame seeds

9 Arrange ¼ of Spicy Tuna in a line at the bottom end of each nori sheet on top of the cauliflower rice. Place ¼ of cucumber on top of each line of Spicy Tuna.

10 Starting with the end where the tuna and cucumber are, roll up each sheet of nori as tightly as you can into a log. Arrange ¼ of avocado slices on top of each sushi roll.

11 Carefully slice each roll into ½"-thick slices.

12 Place sushi slices (standing upright) onto a serving platter. Drizzle on the Spicy Mayonnaise decoratively, and sprinkle on scallion and sesame seeds. Top with Crunchy Onion Topping. Serve.

Per Serving
Calories: 447 | Fat: 36g | Protein: 18g | Sodium: 888mg | Fiber: 4g | Carbohydrates: 9g | Net Carbohydrates: 5g | Sugar: 4g

Chicken Tikka Masala

Takeout from your favorite local Indian restaurant will become a thing of the past once you try this recipe! It's well spiced but not overly hot, and you can adjust the heat level up or down by adding more or less jalapeño and cayenne pepper. The best thing to serve it with? Cauliflower rice, of course!

CHICKEN

**2 tablespoons 5% plain
Greek yogurt**

2 tablespoons fresh lemon juice

**2 medium cloves garlic,
peeled and crushed**

**1/2 tablespoon grated
fresh ginger**

1 teaspoon garam masala

1/2 teaspoon salt

1/4 teaspoon cayenne pepper

**1 1/2 pounds boneless, skinless
chicken thighs, cut into 1" cubes**

1 tablespoon avocado oil

TIKKA MASALA SAUCE

4 tablespoons ghee

**1 medium yellow onion,
peeled and diced**

**6 medium cloves garlic,
peeled and crushed**

**1 tablespoon grated
fresh ginger**

**1 medium jalapeño pepper,
seeded and minced**

2 teaspoons garam masala

1 teaspoon chili powder

1 teaspoon cumin

*Ingredients continued on
the next page* ▶

1 *For the Chicken:* In a large bowl, whisk together yogurt, lemon juice, garlic, ginger, garam masala, salt, and cayenne pepper. Add chicken and stir well to coat chicken.

2 Cover the bowl and refrigerate 2 hours or up to 24 hours.

3 Preheat oven to 425°F. Drizzle oil on a large baking sheet.

4 Spread out chicken on the baking sheet, scraping off excess marinade. Bake until it's fully cooked (it should reach an internal temperature of 165°F and have no pink in the center), about 15–20 minutes, flipping chicken about halfway through the cooking time.

5 *For the Tikka Masala Sauce:* Add ghee to a large, deep skillet over medium heat. Once melted, add onion and cook until it's starting to soften and caramelize in spots, about 3 minutes, stirring occasionally.

6 Add garlic, ginger, and jalapeño and cook 1 minute, stirring constantly.

7 Add garam masala, chili powder, cumin, coriander, paprika, salt, turmeric, black pepper, cayenne pepper, and fenugreek and cook 30 seconds, stirring constantly.

8 Add water and tomato paste and bring to a boil. Turn heat down slightly and let it boil 5 minutes, stirring frequently.

Continued on the next page ▶

TIKKA MASALA SAUCE
(continued)

1 teaspoon coriander

1 teaspoon sweet paprika

¾ teaspoon salt

½ teaspoon turmeric

¼ teaspoon ground black pepper

¼ teaspoon cayenne pepper

¼ teaspoon fenugreek

2 cups water

3 tablespoons tomato paste

½ cup heavy whipping cream

2 tablespoons chopped fresh cilantro, for garnish

9 Remove from heat and stir in cream.

10 *To Serve:* Stir chicken into the sauce. Transfer to a serving dish, sprinkle cilantro on top, and serve.

Per Serving
Calories: 330 | Fat: 23g | Protein: 23g | Sodium: 572mg | Fiber: 2g | Carbohydrates: 7g | Net Carbohydrates: 5g | Sugar: 3g

Crab Rangoon Dip

If you love crab rangoon, you're going to love this dip! We take the best part—the filling—and make it the star of the show. You can use either fresh or canned lump crab for this recipe; just be sure to pick through it to remove any shell fragments before adding it.

8 ounces cream cheese, at room temperature

½ cup mayonnaise

½ cup full-fat sour cream

1 tablespoon fresh lemon juice

1½ teaspoons garlic powder

1 teaspoon onion powder

1 teaspoon Worcestershire sauce

1 teaspoon tamari sauce

¼ teaspoon ground black pepper

3 drops liquid stevia

12 ounces lump crab

1 medium scallion, green and white parts, thinly sliced

1 cup shredded full-fat mozzarella cheese

1 tablespoon minced fresh chives, for garnish

1 Preheat oven to 375°F.

2 In a large bowl, beat together cream cheese, mayonnaise, sour cream, lemon juice, garlic powder, onion powder, Worcestershire sauce, tamari sauce, black pepper, and stevia. Stir in crab and scallion.

3 Spread mixture evenly into a 2-quart casserole dish. Sprinkle mozzarella on top.

4 Bake until the dip is warm throughout and starting to brown in spots on top, about 20–25 minutes.

5 Sprinkle chives on top and serve warm.

Per Serving
Calories: 200 | Fat: 16g | Protein: 9g | Sodium: 382mg | Fiber: 0g | Carbohydrates: 2g | Net Carbohydrates: 2g | Sugar: 1g

What Can You Dip With?

We like to serve this dip with homemade Tortilla Chips (see Chapter 6) or the easy low-carb tortilla chips in our recipe for Chips and Queso (see Chapter 6). Fresh vegetables that are low in carbs are also great, such as celery sticks, green bell pepper slices, or broccoli florets.

Keto Pad Thai

You're only about 30 minutes away from your new favorite pad thai recipe! The balanced flavor profile between salty, sweet, sour, bitter, and umami really sets Thai cuisine apart. In traditional pad thai, tamarind is used for the sour component. However, it's high in carbohydrates, so we omit tamarind and use fresh lime juice here instead.

2 tablespoons avocado oil, divided

2 large eggs, lightly beaten

6 ounces small raw shrimp, peeled and deveined

1/2 small yellow onion, peeled and thinly sliced

1 small carrot, peeled and julienned

2 1/2 cups fresh bean sprouts, divided

3 medium cloves garlic, peeled and crushed

1 teaspoon grated fresh ginger

2 tablespoons tamari sauce

1 tablespoon fresh lime juice

1 1/2 teaspoons keto brown sugar, lightly packed

3/4 teaspoon fish sauce

1/2 teaspoon crushed red pepper flakes

1/8 teaspoon ground white pepper

1 (400-gram) can Palmini hearts of palm linguine, rinsed and drained

1 tablespoon lightly salted peanuts, crushed

3 tablespoons chopped fresh cilantro, for serving

3 lime wedges, for serving

1 Heat a large nonstick skillet over high heat. Once pan is very hot, add 1/2 tablespoon oil and turn heat down to medium-high. Add eggs and scramble to break them up. Let cook until they are set, about 1 minute. Transfer eggs to a small bowl and set aside.

2 To same skillet, add 1 tablespoon oil. Once hot, add shrimp and cook until they turn pink, about 2–3 minutes, stirring occasionally. Transfer shrimp to a medium bowl and set aside.

3 To same skillet, add remaining 1/2 tablespoon oil, onion, carrot, and 2 cups bean sprouts. Turn heat down to medium. Cook until vegetables are just starting to soften, about 1–2 minutes, stirring frequently.

4 Stir in garlic, ginger, tamari sauce, lime juice, brown sugar, fish sauce, red pepper flakes, and white pepper and cook 30 seconds, stirring constantly.

5 Add Palmini linguine and cook 2 minutes, stirring frequently. Stir in scrambled eggs and cooked shrimp. Remove from heat.

6 Top with remaining 1/2 cup bean sprouts, peanuts, and cilantro.

7 Serve each portion along with a lime wedge to squeeze on top.

Per Serving
Calories: 231 | Fat: 14g | Protein: 16g | Sodium: 1,323mg | Fiber: 3g | Carbohydrates: 12g | Net Carbohydrates: 8g | Sugar: 3g

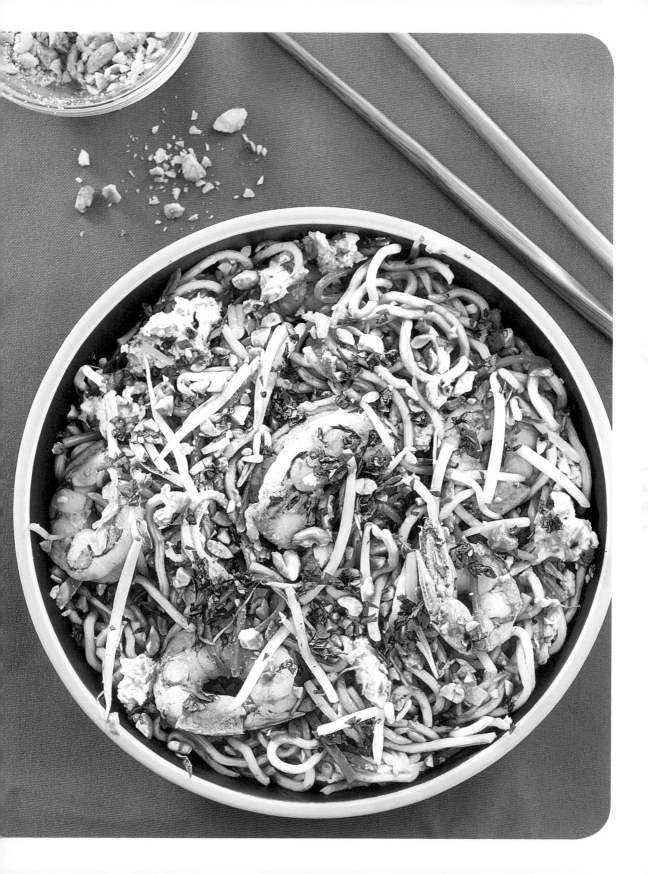

Dan Dan Noodles

Dan Dan Noodles, aka Dan Dan Mian, are perhaps the most famous Sichuan street food. And it's for good reason! The dish features noodles (which we replace with zoodles here) in a complex spicy, savory, and slightly sweet sauce. It comes together faster than you can order takeout from your favorite Asian restaurant!

4 tablespoons coconut oil

1¹/₂ pounds 85% lean ground beef

1 medium yellow onion, peeled and diced

4 large cloves garlic, peeled and crushed

1¹/₂ tablespoons grated fresh ginger

3 tablespoons coconut aminos

2 tablespoons apple cider vinegar

1 tablespoon tahini

1 tablespoon tomato paste

¹/₂ tablespoon sriracha

¹/₄ teaspoon salt

10 drops liquid stevia

1 cup water

1 tablespoon white miso paste

2 medium zucchini, spiralized into noodles

¹/₂ tablespoon sesame seeds

2 medium scallions, green and white parts, thinly sliced

¹/₄ teaspoon crushed red pepper flakes, for garnish

1 To a large, deep skillet over medium-high heat, add oil. Once hot, add ground beef and onion and cook until the meat is browned, about 8 minutes, stirring occasionally.

2 Add garlic and ginger and cook 1 minute more, stirring constantly.

3 Stir in coconut aminos, vinegar, tahini, tomato paste, sriracha, salt, stevia, and water.

4 Bring to a boil, and then cover the skillet, turn heat down to simmer, and cook until thickened, about 10 minutes, stirring occasionally.

5 Turn off heat and stir in miso paste.

6 To serve, top zucchini noodles with the hot meat mixture and sprinkle sesame seeds, scallions, and red pepper flakes on top.

Per Serving
Calories: 330 | Fat: 20g | Protein: 23g | Sodium: 506mg | Fiber: 2g | Carbohydrates: 9g | Net Carbohydrates: 7g | Sugar: 4g

What Is White Miso Paste?

Miso paste is a Japanese seasoning made by fermenting soybeans with a type of mold called koji, as well as salt and other ingredients, including rice, barley, and so on. It adds a rich umami flavor and a lot of complexity. One tablespoon of miso has about 3.5g net carbs, but the good thing is that you don't need a lot because a little goes a long way. You can find different types of miso at Asian grocery stores or online.

Tandoori Chicken

Normally tandoori chicken is cooked in a clay oven called a tandoor. Of course, most of us don't have access to that at home! There are two tricks to making flavorful, moist tandoori chicken in your own kitchen. The first is to marinate it at least 2 hours to tenderize the meat and infuse it with flavor, and the second is to cook it in a fairly hot oven. And if you have a grill, feel free to grill the chicken for an even more authentic flavor!

¼ cup 5% plain Greek yogurt

2 tablespoons fresh lemon juice

2 tablespoons avocado oil, divided

4 medium cloves garlic, peeled and crushed

1 tablespoon grated fresh ginger

1½ teaspoons garam masala

1 teaspoon salt

¾ teaspoon turmeric

¾ teaspoon cumin

¾ teaspoon coriander

¾ teaspoon sweet paprika

¼ teaspoon cayenne pepper

3 pounds chicken drumsticks and thighs, bone-in and skinless

1 In a large bowl, whisk together yogurt, lemon juice, 1 tablespoon oil, garlic, ginger, garam masala, salt, turmeric, cumin, coriander, paprika, and cayenne pepper.

2 Add chicken to the marinade and toss well to coat.

3 Cover the bowl and refrigerate at least 2 hours or up to 24 hours.

4 Preheat oven to 425°F. Drizzle remaining 1 tablespoon oil on a large baking sheet and spread it around.

5 Remove chicken from marinade, scraping off any excess. Arrange chicken on the prepared baking sheet.

6 Bake until chicken is fully cooked and reaches an internal temperature of 165°F, about 50 minutes. Serve.

Per Serving
Calories: 522 | Fat: 23g | Protein: 64g | Sodium: 697mg | Fiber: 0g | Carbohydrates: 4g | Net Carbohydrates: 4g | Sugar: 1g

CHAPTER 6
Taqueria Night

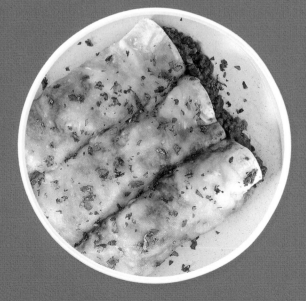

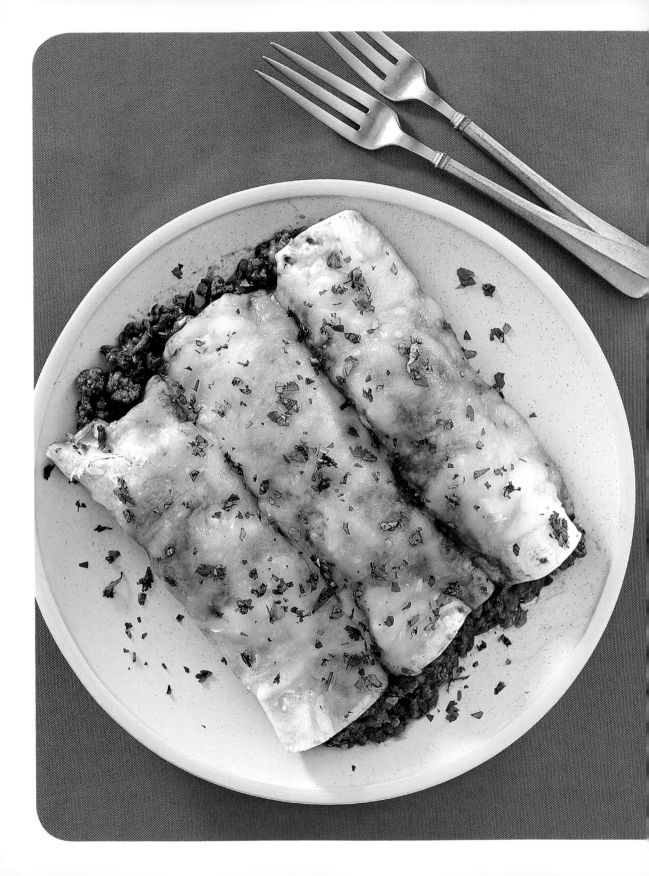

Ground Beef Enchiladas

Gooey melted cheese, seasoned meat, and saucy goodness make enchiladas one of our favorite meals ever. Be sure to look for red enchilada sauce with no sugar added, or make your own. And we think the best way to eat these enchiladas is with a dollop of sour cream on top.

Olive oil spray

4 (6"-8") low-carb tortilla wraps

1 batch Ground Beef Taco Meat (see recipe in this chapter)

½ cup no-sugar-added red enchilada sauce

1 cup pre-shredded Mexican four-cheese blend

2 tablespoons minced fresh cilantro

1 Preheat oven to 375°F. Spray the inside of an 8" × 8" casserole dish with olive oil.

2 Lay tortillas on a flat surface. Divide the taco meat between tortillas, and roll up each as tightly as you can. Place them in the prepared casserole dish, seam-side-down.

3 Spread enchilada sauce on top and sprinkle cheese on top.

4 Bake until enchiladas are warm and the cheese is melted, about 15–20 minutes. If desired, broil a couple minutes to brown the cheese.

5 Serve warm, topped with cilantro.

Per Serving
Calories: 384 | Fat: 19g | Protein: 35g | Sodium: 1,243mg | Fiber: 13g | Carbohydrates: 23g | Net Carbohydrates: 10g | Sugar: 4g

What Other Meat Can You Use?

Leftover shredded chicken is delicious, and so is pulled pork. Check out the Carnitas Tacos (see recipe in this chapter) if you want to go with pork!

SERVES

8,

YIELDS
1¼ CUPS
QUESO
AND 48
CHIPS

Chips and Queso

Chips and dip are a quintessential junk food classic. And what better for dipping than warm, gooey queso?! Instead of using store-bought tortilla wraps to make your own tortilla chips, check out the recipe for Tortilla Chips in this chapter. Or make them both and see which you like better!

CHIPS

6 (6"–8") low-carb tortilla wraps

3 tablespoons extra-virgin olive oil

¼ teaspoon salt

¼ teaspoon ground black pepper

QUESO

4 ounces cream cheese

6 tablespoons heavy whipping cream

6 ounces shredded Cheddar cheese

3 tablespoons no-sugar-added salsa

½ teaspoon onion powder

½ teaspoon garlic powder

¼ teaspoon ground black pepper

⅛ teaspoon chili powder

1/16 teaspoon cayenne pepper

1 *For the Chips:* Preheat oven to 350°F.

2 Cut each tortilla circle into eight wedges and place in a large bowl. Add oil, salt, and black pepper and use your hands to toss together, coating them well.

3 Spread out tortillas evenly on two large baking sheets. Bake until they're golden on both sides, about 15 minutes, flipping them once halfway through the cooking time. The chips will crisp as they cool.

4 *For the Queso:* While the chips bake, make the queso. In a medium saucepan over medium-low heat, whisk together cream cheese and cream. Once smooth, whisk in Cheddar a little at a time until fully incorporated. Add salsa, onion powder, garlic powder, black pepper, chili powder, and cayenne pepper and whisk to combine. Remove from heat, but serve while warm so it's dippable.

5 *To Serve:* Serve chips cool and queso warm.

Per Serving
Calories: 258 | Fat: 20g | Protein: 10g | Sodium: 478mg | Fiber: 8g | Carbohydrates: 13g | Net Carbohydrates: 5g | Sugar: 1g

How to Reheat Queso

If you refrigerate leftovers, this queso will solidify! To get it dippable again, reheat it in a saucepan over low heat on the stovetop, or in a microwave-safe dish in the microwave in 30-second increments.

Loaded Nachos

Next time movie night rolls around, make a batch of Loaded Nachos and get ready for your new favorite movie night food. Instead of the Ground Beef Taco Meat called for here, you can substitute pulled pork if you have any left over from Carnitas Tacos (see recipe in this chapter).

CHIPS

6 (6"-8") low-carb tortilla wraps

3 tablespoons extra-virgin olive oil

¼ teaspoon salt

¼ teaspoon ground black pepper

OTHER

¼ batch Ground Beef Taco Meat (see recipe in this chapter)

6 ounces shredded Cheddar cheese

2 tablespoons pickled jalapeño slices, chopped

1 medium ripe Hass avocado, peeled, pitted, and chopped

¼ cup diced cherry tomatoes

2 tablespoons minced red onion

2 tablespoons minced fresh cilantro

4 tablespoons full-fat sour cream

1 *For the Chips:* Preheat oven to 350°F.

2 Cut each tortilla circle into eight wedges and place in a large bowl. Add oil, salt, and black pepper and use your hands to toss together, coating them well.

3 Spread out tortillas evenly on two large baking sheets. Bake until they're golden on both sides, about 15 minutes, flipping them once halfway through the cooking time. The chips will crisp as they cool.

4 *To Make the Loaded Nachos:* Preheat the broiler.

5 Put all crispy tortilla chips in a pile on one large baking sheet.

6 Dollop Ground Beef Taco Meat around chips and sprinkle Cheddar evenly on top.

7 Broil until cheese is melted, about 3–5 minutes. Stay with it because this can happen fast.

8 Remove from the broiler and sprinkle on jalapeños, avocado, tomatoes, onion, and cilantro. Dollop sour cream on top. Serve immediately.

Per Serving
Calories: 158 | Fat: 11g | Protein: 8g | Sodium: 347mg | Fiber: 7g | Carbohydrates: 10g | Net Carbohydrates: 3g | Sugar: 1g

Taco Salad Bowls

These Taco Salad Bowls deliver big in terms of flavor and texture. Feel free to customize them to suit your taste preferences with your favorite taco salad components. Sliced black olives are one of our favorite additions!

8 cups baby spinach leaves

1 batch Ground Beef Taco Meat (see recipe in this chapter)

¼ cup chopped tomatoes

1 medium ripe Hass avocado, peeled, pitted, and chopped

4 tablespoons no-sugar-added salsa

4 tablespoons full-fat sour cream

2 tablespoons minced red onion

2 Crispy Taco Shells, coarsely crunched up (see recipe in this chapter)

1 Divide spinach leaves between four shallow bowls.

2 Top each with ¼ of Ground Beef Taco Meat, tomatoes, and avocado.

3 On each, dollop 1 tablespoon salsa and 1 tablespoon sour cream. Sprinkle on ½ tablespoon onion and ¼ of the crunched-up Crispy Taco Shells. Serve immediately.

Per Serving
Calories: 439 | Fat: 26g | Protein: 32g | Sodium: 851mg | Fiber: 5g | Carbohydrates: 12g | Net Carbohydrates: 7g | Sugar: 4g

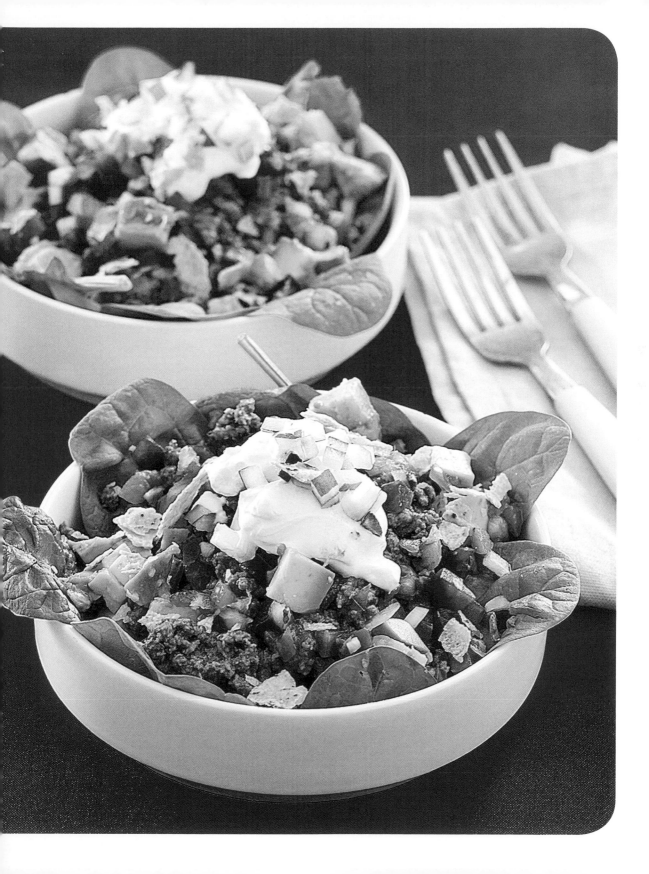

Ground Beef Taco Meat

When you have a good base recipe for taco meat there are a ton of easy recipes you can make, which makes this dish perfect for meal prep! Make a double batch on the weekend and use it to make easy dinners during the week. You can use this to make Ground Beef Enchiladas, Loaded Nachos, Taco Salad Bowls (see recipes in this chapter), and more!

1 pound 85% lean ground beef

½ medium yellow onion, peeled and diced

2 medium cloves garlic, peeled and minced

2 teaspoons chili powder

½ tablespoon cumin

1 teaspoon dried oregano

¾ teaspoon salt

¼ teaspoon ground black pepper

⅛ teaspoon cayenne pepper

2 tablespoons tomato paste

½ cup water

1 To a large skillet over medium-high heat, add ground beef, onion, and garlic. Cook until beef is browned and onion is softened, about 8 minutes, stirring occasionally.

2 Stir in chili powder, cumin, oregano, salt, black pepper, and cayenne pepper and cook 30 seconds, stirring constantly.

3 Add tomato paste and water and stir to combine. Cook until water cooks off and mixture thickens, about 5 minutes, stirring frequently.

4 Serve or store in an airtight container in the refrigerator up to 3 days.

Per Serving
Calories: 222 | Fat: 10g | Protein: 23g | Sodium: 609mg | Fiber: 2g | Carbohydrates: 5g | Net Carbohydrates: 3g | Sugar: 2g

Chicken Fajitas

The beauty of these Chicken Fajitas is that they're not only a quick and healthy weeknight dinner but also a good way to use up leftover chicken! Or to help this recipe come together quick, pick up a rotisserie chicken on your way home from work.

CHICKEN AND VEGETABLE FAJITA MIX

2 tablespoons avocado oil

1 pound boneless, skinless chicken thighs, thinly sliced

½ medium yellow onion, peeled and thinly sliced

½ medium green bell pepper, seeded and thinly sliced

½ medium red bell pepper, seeded and thinly sliced

3 medium cloves garlic, peeled and minced

1 teaspoon chili powder

1 teaspoon cumin

½ teaspoon dried oregano

¾ teaspoon salt

¼ teaspoon ground black pepper

⅛ teaspoon cayenne pepper

OTHER

4 (6"-8") low-carb tortilla wraps

4 tablespoons full-fat sour cream

1 medium lime, cut into 4 wedges, for squeezing on top

1 *For the Chicken and Vegetable Fajita Mix:* To a large, deep skillet over medium-high heat, add oil. Once hot, add chicken and cook until starting to brown in places, about 5 minutes.

2 Stir in onion, green bell pepper, and red bell pepper and cook until the chicken is fully cooked and vegetables are slightly softened, about 5 minutes, stirring occasionally.

3 Turn heat down to medium-low. Add garlic, chili powder, cumin, oregano, salt, black pepper, and cayenne pepper and cook 2 minutes, stirring constantly. Remove from heat.

4 *To Serve:* Divide chicken fajita mixture between tortillas and dollop 1 tablespoon sour cream on top of each. Serve each with 1 lime wedge to squeeze on top.

Per Serving
Calories: 303 | Fat: 17g | Protein: 27g | Sodium: 808mg | Fiber: 12g | Carbohydrates: 20g | Net Carbohydrates: 8g | Sugar: 2g

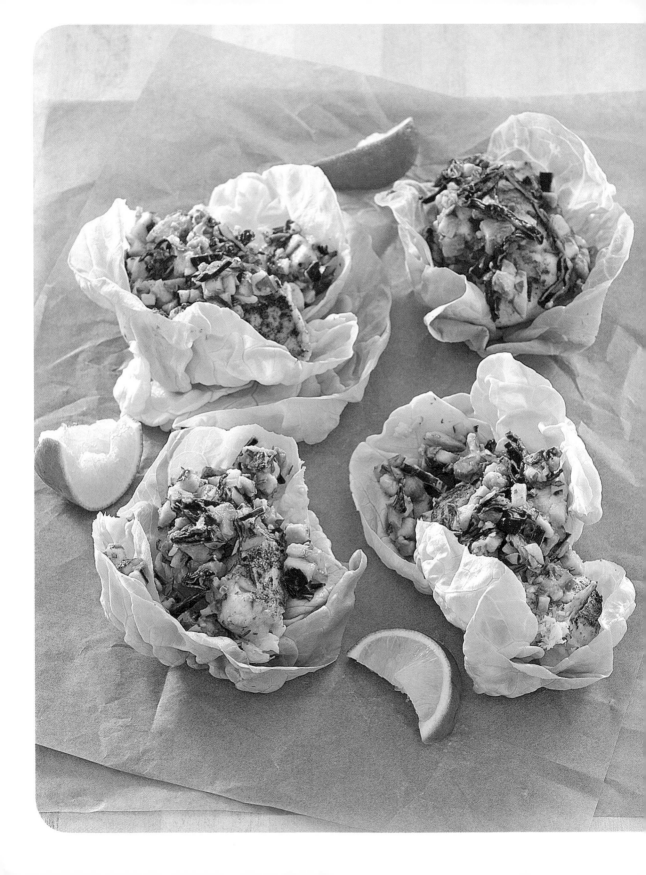

Fish Tacos

We like our Fish Tacos full of fresh, bright flavor! The quick slaw is an easy way to pack in flavor and nutrition, and it also makes these tacos a filling meal. If you can fit it in your macros, we love adding a little bit of fresh orange segments to the slaw to bump up the citrus flavor.

FISH

4 (6-ounce) cod fillets
¾ teaspoon salt
½ teaspoon chili powder
½ teaspoon cumin
½ teaspoon garlic powder
½ teaspoon dried thyme
¼ teaspoon ground black pepper
2 tablespoons avocado oil

OTHER

1 medium ripe Hass avocado, peeled, pitted, and diced
1 cup thinly sliced red cabbage
¼ cup minced red onion
¼ cup chopped fresh cilantro
½ medium jalapeño, minced
2 tablespoons fresh lime juice
2 tablespoons avocado oil
¼ teaspoon salt
8 leaves Bibb lettuce

1 *For the Fish:* Pat fillets dry with paper towels. Place fillets on a cutting board and season both sides with salt, chili powder, cumin, garlic powder, thyme, and black pepper.

2 To a large nonstick skillet over medium-high heat, add oil. Once hot, add fish and cook until browned on both sides and opaque in the center, about 4–5 minutes on the first side and 2–4 minutes on the second side.

3 Remove skillet from heat and drape a piece of foil over the top. Let fish sit like this 3 minutes.

4 *To Serve:* In a medium bowl, gently stir together avocado, cabbage, onion, cilantro, jalapeño, lime juice, oil, and salt.

5 Cut each fillet in half. Lay lettuce leaves on a work surface and place ½ fillet in each leaf. Divide avocado mixture between the lettuce leaves. Serve immediately, folding lettuce leaves up like a taco shell to eat.

Per Serving
Calories: 314 | Fat: 19g | Protein: 27g | Sodium: 1,405mg | Fiber: 3g | Carbohydrates: 7g | Net Carbohydrates: 4g | Sugar: 2g

Carnitas Tacos

Carnitas ("little meats") is a Mexican dish of tender, juicy shredded pork that's scrumptious served up as tacos! Instead of using tortilla wraps for this, it's also delicious served as lettuce tacos, using large lettuce leaves as the tortillas.

CARNITAS

1 (4-pound) pork butt

1¼ teaspoons salt

1 teaspoon ground black pepper

1 teaspoon chili powder

1 teaspoon cumin

1 teaspoon garlic powder

1 teaspoon onion powder

¼ teaspoon cayenne pepper

OTHER

6 (6"-8") low-carb tortilla wraps

6 tablespoons minced white onion

6 tablespoons chopped fresh cilantro

6 tablespoons no-sugar-added salsa

1½ medium limes, cut into 6 wedges, for squeezing on top

1 *For the Carnitas:* Place pork on a cutting board and rub both sides with salt, black pepper, chili powder, cumin, garlic powder, onion powder, and cayenne pepper.

2 Wrap pork in plastic wrap and refrigerate at least 2 hours or up to 12 hours.

3 Preheat oven to 325°F. Unwrap pork and discard the plastic wrap. Place pork on a roasting rack inside a roasting pan.

4 Roast until pork reaches an internal temperature of 190°F, about 3–4 hours.

5 Remove pork from oven, place a piece of foil on top, and let it rest 30 minutes before using two forks to shred it.

6 *To Serve:* Divide shredded pork between tortillas and top each with 1 tablespoon onion, 1 tablespoon cilantro, and 1 tablespoon salsa. Serve each with 1 lime wedge to squeeze on top.

Per Serving
Calories: 543 | Fat: 31g | Protein: 52g | Sodium: 1,057mg | Fiber: 12g | Carbohydrates: 18g | Net Carbohydrates: 6g | Sugar: 1g

What Is Pork Butt?

It's a bit of a misnomer because pork butt is from the shoulder area of the pig. You can find it labeled Boston butt.

Chicken Burrito Bowls

The trick to this recipe is to make a double batch of Chicken and Vegetable Fajita Mix (from the Chicken Fajitas recipe in this chapter) so that you can have fajitas one night and burrito bowls the next. And sometimes we like to switch it up with flank steak instead of boneless, skinless chicken thighs!

1 batch Chicken and Vegetable Fajita Mix, warm (see Chicken Fajitas recipe in this chapter)

1 cup riced cauliflower

1 medium ripe Hass avocado, peeled, pitted, and quartered

4 tablespoons no-sugar-added salsa

4 tablespoons crumbled queso fresco

4 tablespoons chopped fresh cilantro

1 medium lime, cut into 4 wedges, for squeezing on top

1 Divide Chicken and Vegetable Fajita Mix between four serving bowls.

2 Top each with ¼ cup cauliflower, ¼ avocado, 1 tablespoon salsa, 1 tablespoon queso fresco, and 1 tablespoon cilantro.

3 Serve each with 1 lime wedge to squeeze on top.

Per Serving
Calories: 319 | Fat: 19g | Protein: 24g | Sodium: 592mg | Fiber: 4g | Carbohydrates: 10g | Net Carbohydrates: 6g | Sugar: 3g

Portobello Mushroom Fajitas

A question we get asked a lot is if it's possible to eat vegetarian on keto. The answer is yes! Actually, vegan keto is possible as well. This recipe is vegetarian, and it makes great use of umami-rich portobello mushrooms.

2 tablespoons avocado oil

2 tablespoons unsalted butter

1½ pounds portobello mushrooms, sliced into ¾"-thick slices

½ medium yellow onion, peeled and thinly sliced

½ medium red bell pepper, seeded and thinly sliced

3 medium cloves garlic, peeled and minced

1 teaspoon chili powder

1 teaspoon cumin

½ teaspoon dried oregano

½ teaspoon salt

¼ teaspoon ground black pepper

⅛ teaspoon cayenne pepper

1 tablespoon coconut aminos

4 (6"-8") low-carb tortilla wraps

1 medium ripe Hass avocado, peeled, pitted, and diced

½ cup crumbled queso fresco

4 tablespoons chopped fresh cilantro

1 medium lime, cut into 4 wedges

1. In a large, deep skillet over medium to medium-high heat, heat oil and butter. Once hot, add portobello slices and cook until starting to soften, about 3–5 minutes.

2. Stir in onion and bell pepper and cook until vegetables are slightly softened, about 5 minutes, stirring occasionally.

3. Turn heat down to medium-low. Add garlic, chili powder, cumin, oregano, salt, black pepper, cayenne pepper, and coconut aminos and cook 2 minutes, stirring constantly. Remove from heat.

4. Divide portobello mixture between tortillas and top each with ¼ of avocado, 2 tablespoons queso fresco, and 1 tablespoon cilantro. Serve each with 1 lime wedge to squeeze on top.

Per Serving
Calories: 323 | Fat: 22g | Protein: 13g | Sodium: 810mg | Fiber: 17g | Carbohydrates: 29g | Net Carbohydrates: 12g | Sugar: 6g

What Is Coconut Aminos?

Coconut aminos is a fermented savory sauce that's made from coconut palm sap. It has a salty, umami flavor that's similar to soy sauce or tamari sauce. In this recipe, it adds great depth of flavor and pairs well with the portobello mushrooms.

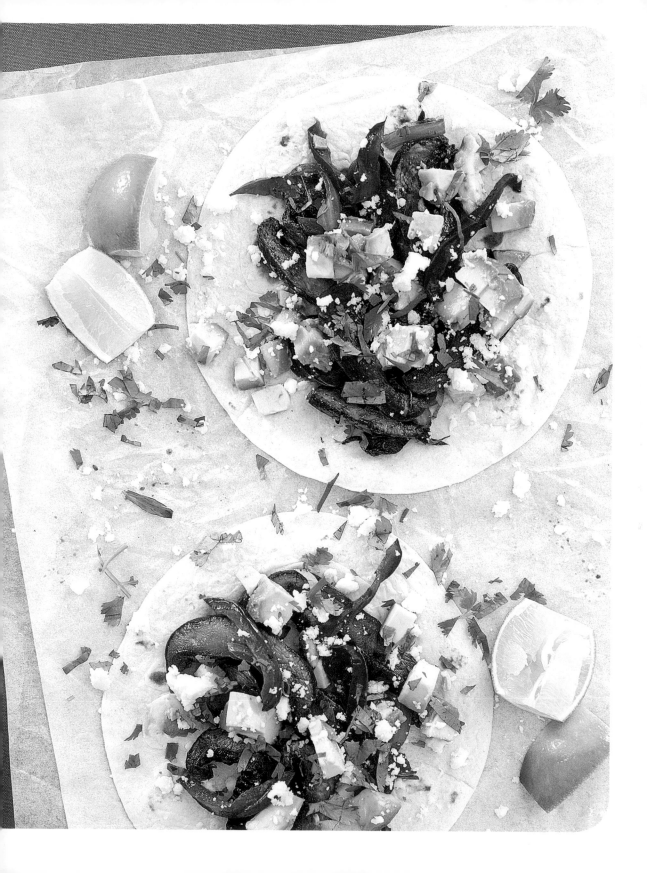

7-Layer Dip

This dip is seven layers of taco-style bliss. And because every good dip needs a dipper, we recommend whipping up a batch (or three) of our Tortilla Chips to serve with it (see recipe in this chapter).

1 batch Ground Beef Taco Meat, cooled (see recipe in this chapter)

2 cups full-fat sour cream

2 medium ripe Hass avocados, peeled, pitted, and chopped

1 tablespoon fresh lime juice

8 ounces shredded Cheddar cheese

1 cup chopped tomatoes

2 (2.25-ounce) cans sliced black olives, drained and patted dry

3 medium scallions, green and white parts, thinly sliced

1 Spread Ground Beef Taco Meat evenly in the bottom of a 3-quart casserole dish.

2 Dollop sour cream on top of meat, and then spread it out evenly.

3 Sprinkle avocado on top of sour cream. Squeeze lime juice on top of avocado.

4 Spread Cheddar on top of avocado.

5 Sprinkle tomatoes evenly on top, and then olives and scallions.

6 Serve chilled, or store it covered in the refrigerator up to 3 days before serving.

Per Serving
Calories: 229 | Fat: 17g | Protein: 11g | Sodium: 345mg | Fiber: 2g | Carbohydrates: 5g | Net Carbohydrates: 3g | Sugar: 2g

Tortilla Chips

Crispy, crunchy tortilla chips are an integral part of every junk food repertoire. And they're versatile; eat them with queso, salsa, or guacamole! You can easily play with the flavor profile to suit your tastes by adding different spices such as onion powder, garlic powder, chili powder, paprika, cayenne, and so on.

1½ cups pre-shredded low-moisture part-skim mozzarella

½ cup almond flour

1 tablespoon golden flaxseed meal

¼ teaspoon salt

⅛ teaspoon ground black pepper

1 Preheat oven to 375°F. Line two large baking sheets with parchment paper or Silpat liners.

2 Melt cheese in a double boiler or microwave. If you're using the microwave, place cheese in a large microwave-safe bowl, microwave it 1 minute, and then in 15-second intervals after that, checking and stirring until it's melted.

3 Once cheese is melted, use a fork to mix in almond flour, flaxseed meal, salt, and black pepper. Use your hands to knead it a bit until it looks like dough. (If dough cools too much, you may need to microwave it for a few seconds so it's easier to work with.)

4 Divide dough into two equal balls. Spread or roll out each ball of dough onto the prepared baking sheets until each is a rectangle about 8" × 10". Cut each into square- or triangle-shaped chips. Spread the chips on the baking sheets so they're not touching.

5 Bake until golden brown on both sides, about 10–15 minutes, flipping chips once halfway through the cooking time. Serve.

Per Serving
Calories: 149 | Fat: 11g | Protein: 8g | Sodium: 272mg | Fiber: 1g | Carbohydrates: 3g | Net Carbohydrates: 2g | Sugar: 1g

Can You Make These Tortilla Chips Ahead of Time?

Yes! Store the chips up to 3 days in an airtight container at room temperature. To recrisp the chips after the first day, bake them for 5 minutes at 350°F.

Crispy Taco Shells

Sometimes you want a soft tortilla shell, but sometimes nothing less than a crispy shell will do! It's that crunch factor that we're going for here. You can fill them with anything you'd put in a taco, or use them to make Taco Salad Bowls (see recipe in this chapter).

2 cups pre-shredded Cheddar cheese

1 Drape a long wooden spoon over two tall glasses.

2 Heat a 6" nonstick skillet over medium heat for 2 minutes.

3 Sprinkle ½ cup cheese evenly in the bottom of the skillet. Cook 2 minutes.

4 Remove from heat for 30 seconds. Use a thin metal spatula to carefully flip cheese.

5 Return skillet to heat and cook 45 seconds.

6 Immediately use the metal spatula to remove cheese and drape it over the wooden spoon to form it into a taco shell. Let it cool.

7 Repeat three more times with remaining cheese. Use these shells any way you'd use crispy taco shells.

Per Serving
Calories: 229 | Fat: 17g | Protein: 14g | Sodium: 363mg | Fiber: 0g | Carbohydrates: 1g | Net Carbohydrates: 1g | Sugar: 0g

How to Make Crispy Taco Shells in the Oven

Preheat oven to 375°F. Line two half-sheet pans (18" × 13") with parchment paper. Measure three (⅓-cup) piles pre-shredded Cheddar cheese onto each pan, spacing them apart to leave room for spreading. Bake one pan at a time until cheese is melted and starting to brown on the edges, about 5–8 minutes. Remove from oven and let cheese sit 1 minute. Use a thin metal spatula to remove cheese circles from pan and drape them over a wooden spoon placed over two tall glasses until cool.

CHAPTER 7

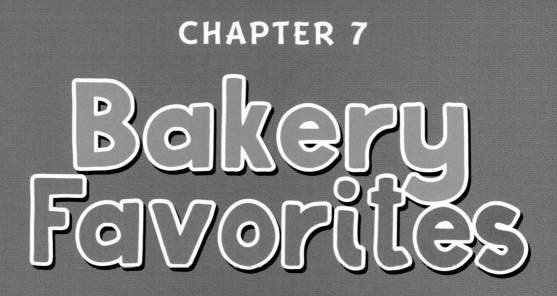

Bakery Favorites

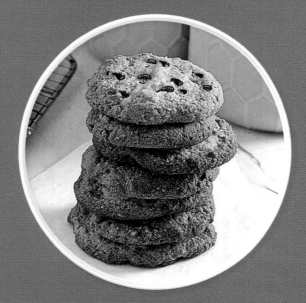

Brownie Bites

Incredibly rich, fudgy, and decadent brownies take a dip in a warm chocolate bath. We like to sprinkle a few toasted slivered almonds on top for crunch and nutty flavor, but shredded coconut is also delicious.

6 tablespoons unsalted butter

8 ounces 90% cocoa dark chocolate, divided

6 tablespoons granulated (or crystalized) allulose sweetener

1 large egg

1 large egg yolk

1 teaspoon pure vanilla extract

1/4 cup almond flour

2 1/2 tablespoons unsweetened cocoa powder

1/4 teaspoon baking powder

1/8 teaspoon salt

10 teaspoons toasted slivered almonds

1 Preheat oven to 350°F. Line a 7 3/4" × 4 1/2" glass loaf pan with parchment paper.

2 In a microwave-safe bowl or double boiler, melt together butter and 2 ounces dark chocolate. Whisk in allulose. Cool slightly, and then whisk in egg, egg yolk, and vanilla.

3 Whisk in almond flour, cocoa powder, baking powder, and salt to combine.

4 Pour batter into the prepared loaf pan. Bake until brownies are set along the outside but still a touch doughy in the center, about 20 minutes. Cool completely.

5 Once brownies are cooled, cut them into ten squares. Freeze brownie squares 15 minutes.

6 In a microwave-safe bowl or double boiler, melt remaining 6 ounces dark chocolate. Dip each brownie square in melted chocolate, let excess drip off, and place on a wax paper–lined baking sheet. Sprinkle 1 teaspoon slivered almonds on top of each before chocolate sets.

7 Let chocolate set before serving. Store in an airtight container in the refrigerator up to 2 weeks.

Per Serving
Calories: 246 | Fat: 23g | Protein: 5g | Sodium: 55mg | Fiber: 4g | Carbohydrates: 16g | Net Carbohydrates: 5g | Sugar: 2g

Edible Cookie Dough

This is basically a cookie dough–flavored fat bomb, so there are no eggs in sight. And if you're wondering: No, this dough can't be baked into cookies; it's meant to be eaten raw.

SERVES 2, YIELDS ABOUT 1/2 CUP

1 ounce cream cheese, at room temperature

1 tablespoon unsalted butter, at room temperature

1/2 tablespoon keto brown sugar

1/2 tablespoon granulated (or crystalized) allulose sweetener

1/2 teaspoon pure vanilla extract

3 tablespoons almond flour

1 teaspoon coconut flour

1/16 teaspoon salt

1/16 teaspoon baking soda

2 tablespoons stevia-sweetened chocolate chips

1 In a small bowl, stir together cream cheese, butter, brown sugar, allulose, vanilla, almond flour, coconut flour, salt, and baking soda until smooth. Stir in chocolate chips.

2 Serve, or store in an airtight container in the refrigerator up to 5 days before serving and let it sit at room temperature for 15 minutes to soften before serving.

Per Serving
Calories: 224 | Fat: 20g | Protein: 4g | Sodium: 164mg | Fiber: 6g | Carbohydrates: 18g | Net Carbohydrates: 3g | Sugar: 1g | Sugar Alcohol: 12g

Chocolate Chip Cookies

If soft chocolate chippers call to you, meet your new favorite keto recipe. These cookies have everything a great chocolate chip cookie should have: rich, buttery flavor with notes of caramel and a hint of vanilla; soft interior; and slightly crispy exterior.

½ cup unsalted butter, slightly softened

¼ cup keto brown sugar

¼ cup granulated (or crystalized) allulose sweetener

1 large egg

1½ teaspoons pure vanilla extract

2 cups almond flour

1½ tablespoons coconut flour

½ teaspoon salt

¼ teaspoon psyllium husk powder

¼ teaspoon baking soda

¾ cup stevia-sweetened chocolate chips

1 Preheat oven to 325°F. Line two large baking sheets with parchment paper or Silpat liners.

2 In a large mixing bowl, cream together butter, brown sugar, allulose, egg, and vanilla.

3 Stir in almond flour, coconut flour, salt, psyllium husk powder, and baking soda. Stir in chocolate chips.

4 Cover bowl with plastic wrap and let dough sit at room temperature 15 minutes.

5 Use a tablespoon-sized scoop to measure dough. Roll dough into balls and arrange them 1"–2" apart on the prepared baking sheet. Lightly flatten each cookie because they don't spread too much on their own.

6 Bake cookies one sheet at a time until they're golden along the outside, about 10–12 minutes.

7 Let cookies cool 10 minutes on sheet before transferring to a wire rack to finish cooling. Bake remaining cookies the same way.

8 Store in an airtight container at room temperature up to 1 week.

Per Serving (Serving size: 4 cookies)
Calories: 333 | Fat: 29g | Protein: 8g | Sodium: 109mg | Fiber: 8g | Carbohydrates: 28g | Net Carbohydrates: 1g | Sugar: 1g | Sugar Alcohol: 17g

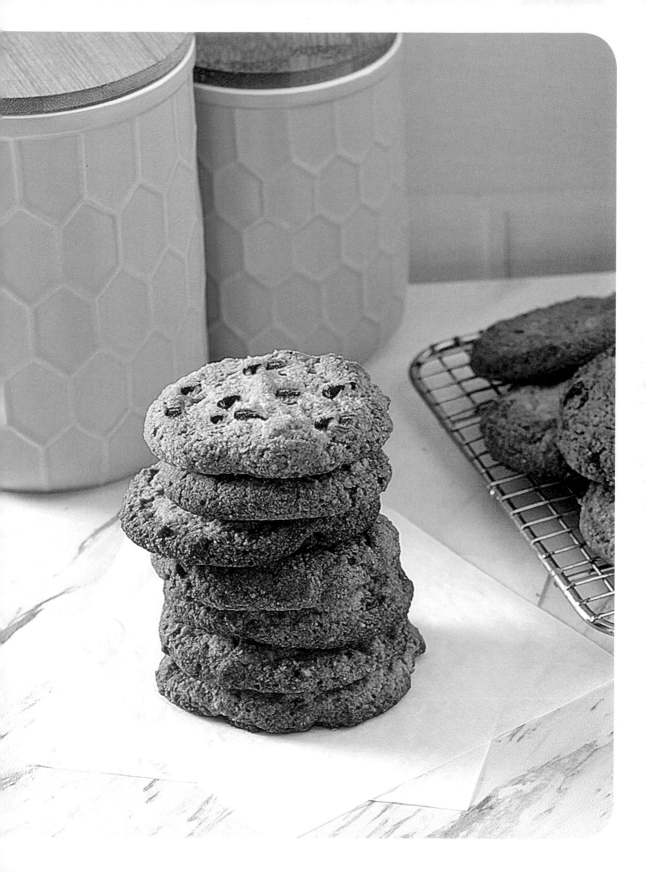

Basic Vanilla Cake

Let's be honest; there's nothing basic about this Basic Vanilla Cake! But you can use it as the base for a bunch of different recipes, including Cake Pops and Tiramisu Parfait (see recipes in this chapter). Or go classic and frost it with our Basic Buttercream (see recipe in this chapter).

Coconut oil spray

12 tablespoons unsalted butter, at room temperature

2/3 cup granulated (or crystalized) allulose sweetener

3 large eggs

1/4 cup whole milk

1 tablespoon pure vanilla extract

1/2 teaspoon apple cider vinegar

1/2 teaspoon liquid stevia

1/4 teaspoon almond extract

2 cups almond flour

1/4 cup golden flaxseed meal

3 tablespoons tapioca flour

2 teaspoons baking powder

3/4 teaspoon salt

1/2 teaspoon psyllium husk powder

1 Preheat oven to 350°F. Spray the inside of a 9" round cake pan with coconut oil. Place a piece of parchment paper that's been trimmed to fit in the bottom of the pan.

2 In a large bowl, cream together butter and allulose, and then beat in eggs, milk, vanilla, vinegar, stevia, and almond extract. The batter will look lumpy and curdled at this point.

3 Beat in almond flour, flaxseed meal, tapioca flour, baking powder, salt, and psyllium husk powder to combine. The batter will be thick.

4 Immediately transfer batter to the prepared cake pan and spread it out evenly. Let batter rest 2 minutes to thicken.

5 Bake until cake is golden and a toothpick inserted in the center comes out clean, about 35 minutes.

6 Run a paring knife along the outside of cake to loosen it from the pan. Turn cake out onto a wire rack and peel the parchment paper off the bottom. Serve.

Per Serving
Calories: 268 | Fat: 23g | Protein: 6g | Sodium: 248mg | Fiber: 3g | Carbohydrates: 17g | Net Carbohydrates: 3g | Sugar: 1g

Can You Switch Up the Flavor of This Cake?

Yes! One of the things we love most about this cake is its flavor versatility. Add a splash of your favorite extract (start with 1/4 teaspoon and go up from there to suit your taste preference) to easily change the flavor profile. A couple of our favorites are lemon extract and peanut butter extract. You can find extracts in a variety of flavors near the vanilla in the grocery store.

Basic Buttercream

This is the keto version of American-style buttercream. You whip together butter, vanilla, keto powdered sweetener, and a couple other things and it's almost instant buttercream! This recipe makes enough to generously frost any 9" round cake.

½ cup unsalted butter, at room temperature

1 teaspoon pure vanilla extract

½ teaspoon vanilla bean paste

⅛ teaspoon salt

2 cups powdered allulose sweetener

2 tablespoons heavy whipping cream

1 In a medium bowl, cream butter with a handheld electric mixer or stand electric mixer. Beat in vanilla extract, vanilla bean paste, and salt.

2 Beat in powdered allulose and then cream until smooth and creamy. It's now ready to frost.

Per Recipe
Calories: 935 | Fat: 96g | Protein: 2g | Sodium: 313mg | Fiber: 0g | Carbohydrates: 290g | Net Carbohydrates: 2g | Sugar: 2g

Can This Buttercream Be Made Ahead of Time?

Yes! You can make this up to 1 week ahead and store it in an airtight container in the refrigerator. When you want to use it, let it sit at room temperature for 15 minutes, and then beat it with a handheld electric mixer until smooth.

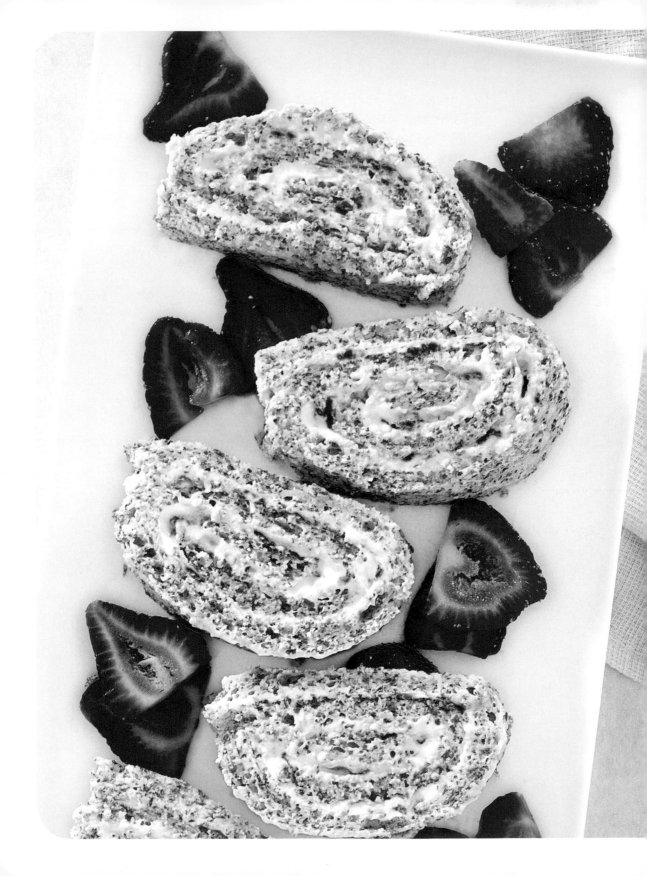

Strawberry Shortcake Cake Roll

This show-stoppingly gorgeous cake roll is a quintessential summer dessert if ever there was one! It's like strawberry shortcake, only better, and without the carbs. It's the perfect treat for a special holiday or any day in between.

SPONGE CAKE

Coconut oil spray, for the pan

¾ cup almond flour

½ cup golden flaxseed meal

2 teaspoons baking powder

¼ teaspoon salt

6 large eggs

½ cup powdered allulose-monk fruit blend sweetener

¼ cup whole milk

1 tablespoon pure vanilla extract

¼ teaspoon almond extract

STRAWBERRY JAM

2 cups frozen strawberries (unthawed)

¼ cup powdered allulose-monk fruit blend sweetener

7 drops liquid stevia

¹⁄₁₆ teaspoon salt

CHEESECAKE BUTTERCREAM

6 ounces cream cheese, softened

6 tablespoons unsalted butter, softened

2 tablespoons powdered allulose-monk fruit blend sweetener

1 teaspoon vanilla bean paste

7 drops liquid stevia

1 *For the Sponge Cake:* Preheat oven to 350°F. Place a piece of parchment paper that's been trimmed to fit in the bottom of a half-sheet pan (18" × 13" × 1"). Spray the sides of the pan and the top of the piece of parchment paper with coconut oil.

2 In a medium bowl, add almond flour, flaxseed meal, baking powder, and salt and whisk to combine. Set aside.

3 Separate egg yolks from egg whites, putting each into separate large bowls.

4 Use a handheld electric mixer to beat egg whites to stiff peaks. Set aside.

5 To the bowl with egg yolks, beat in powdered allulose–monk fruit, milk, vanilla, and almond extract. Once combined, add the dry ingredients and beat to combine.

6 Add ¼ of egg whites to batter and beat well to combine. Add remaining ¾ of egg whites to batter ¼ at a time, folding it in with a rubber spatula to try not to deflate egg whites too much.

7 Pour batter onto the prepared pan and spread it out evenly.

8 Bake until the cake is golden and a toothpick inserted in the center comes out clean, about 10–12 minutes.

9 Turn cake out onto a clean tea towel and peel off parchment paper. Starting at one of the short ends, roll cake up into a log.

Continued on the next page ▶

10 Transfer cake log to a wire rack to cool completely, about 1–2 hours.

11 *For the Strawberry Jam:* In a medium saucepan over medium heat, add all ingredients. Cover saucepan and cook 7 minutes. Use a fork or potato masher to carefully mash berries.

12 Continue cooking uncovered until sauce is thickened, about 3 minutes more, stirring constantly. You should end up with about ¾ cup of jam.

13 Cool to room temperature and then refrigerate to chill.

14 *For the Cheesecake Buttercream:* In a large bowl, add all ingredients and use a handheld electric mixer to beat until smooth and creamy. Refrigerate to chill slightly, about 45 minutes to 1 hour.

15 *To Assemble the Cake:* Carefully unroll cake. Spread Cheesecake Buttercream on the interior, leaving about a 1" gap along the outside. Spread Strawberry Jam on top of buttercream.

16 Tightly roll cake back up the same way it was rolled in the tea towel. Wrap cake roll in plastic wrap and refrigerate 12 hours.

17 Slice cake roll and serve.

Per Serving
Calories: 222 | Fat: 17g | Protein: 7g | Sodium: 232mg | Fiber: 2g | Carbohydrates: 17g | Net Carbohydrates: 4g | Sugar: 3g

Can This Jam Be Used Like Regular Jam?

Yes! Feel free to spread this on keto toast or make it into keto almond butter and jelly sammies. Store this jam in an airtight container in the refrigerator up to 10 days.

SERVES

10,

YIELDS

1 (7")

CHEESE-

CAKE

Classic Cheesecake

You'll be surprised by how great a cheesecake you can whip up right in your own kitchen, even if you don't have any baking experience! Don't let the water bath intimidate you; we use a 9" × 13" casserole dish with a little hot water in the bottom. If you remember to wrap foil around the outside of your springform pan, you should be just fine!

OTHER
Coconut oil spray

CRUST
1¼ cups almond flour

1 tablespoon powdered erythritol

½ teaspoon ground cinnamon

¼ teaspoon salt

4 tablespoons unsalted butter, melted

7 drops liquid stevia

FILLING
2 (8-ounce) blocks full-fat cream cheese, slightly softened

½ cup full-fat sour cream

2 large eggs

¼ cup powdered erythritol

2 teaspoons pure vanilla extract

1 teaspoon fresh lemon juice

¼ teaspoon stevia glycerite

1 Preheat oven to 325°F. Wrap the outside of a 7" springform pan with foil so that it goes about 2" up the sides. Line the bottom of the pan with parchment paper that has been trimmed to fit. Lightly spray the paper and inside of the pan with coconut oil.

2 *For the Crust:* In a medium bowl, use a fork to combine almond flour, powdered erythritol, cinnamon, and salt. Add melted butter and liquid stevia and mix until crumbly. Press this mixture into the bottom and about 1½" up the sides of the prepared pan.

3 *For the Filling:* In a large mixing bowl, use a stand mixer or a handheld electric mixer to beat together all ingredients. Pour filling into crust.

4 Place cheesecake into a 9" × 13" casserole dish. Carefully fill dish with about 1"–1½" of boiling water to create a water bath around the cheesecake.

5 Bake until cheesecake is set along the outside but still jiggly in the center, about 50–60 minutes. Carefully remove cheesecake from the water bath and place it on a wire rack.

6 Cool to room temperature, and then refrigerate to chill, about 4 hours, before slicing and serving.

7 Store covered in the refrigerator up to 10 days.

Per Serving
Calories: 325 | Fat: 28g | Protein: 7g | Sodium: 243mg | Fiber: 2g | Carbohydrates: 10g | Net Carbohydrates: 3g | Sugar: 2g | Sugar Alcohol: 5g

SERVES

16,

YIELDS 1
(2-LAYER)
9" ROUND
CAKE

Quadruple Chocolate Cake

This cake gives you four different doses of chocolate: (1) cocoa powder, (2) mini chocolate chips, (3) chocolate ganache, and (4) chocolate shavings on top. It's a dream come true for any chocolate lover!

FOR THE PANS

2 teaspoons coconut oil

4 teaspoons coconut flour

Coconut oil spray

CHOCOLATE CAKE

2 cups almond flour

¾ cup unsweetened cocoa powder

¼ cup golden flaxseed meal

2 teaspoons baking powder

½ teaspoon salt

¼ teaspoon baking soda

12 tablespoons unsalted butter, slightly softened

1 cup granulated (or crystalized) allulose sweetener

4 large eggs

¾ cup whole milk

1 tablespoon pure vanilla extract

1 teaspoon instant espresso powder, dissolved in 2 teaspoons hot water

1 cup stevia-sweetened mini dark chocolate chips

1 *For the Chocolate Cake:* Preheat oven to 350°F.

2 Rub coconut oil inside two 9" round cake pans. Dust with coconut flour and shake it around inside the pans to coat. Place a piece of parchment paper that's been trimmed to fit inside the bottom of each pan and lightly spray the paper with coconut oil.

3 In a large bowl, whisk together almond flour, cocoa powder, flaxseed meal, baking powder, salt, and baking soda and set aside.

4 In separate large bowl, beat together butter and allulose and then beat in eggs, milk, vanilla, and dissolved espresso.

5 Beat dry ingredients into the wet just until combined. Stir in chocolate chips.

6 Divide batter between the two prepared cake pans, spreading it out evenly.

7 Bake until a toothpick inserted in the center comes out with just a couple crumbs, about 30 minutes, rotating the pans once halfway through the cooking time.

8 Cool cakes 30 minutes in the pans, and then turn them out onto wire racks to finish cooling. Let the cakes cool completely before frosting.

9 *For the Fudgy Ganache:* In a microwave-safe bowl or double boiler, melt together dark chocolate and butter.

10 Whisk in all remaining ingredients. Cool to room temperature, and then frost the cake.

FUDGY GANACHE

2 ounces 90% cocoa dark chocolate

4 tablespoons unsalted butter

¼ cup heavy whipping cream

20 drops liquid stevia

½ teaspoon pure vanilla extract

¹⁄₁₆ teaspoon salt

2 tablespoons powdered erythritol

OTHER

¼ cup 90% cocoa dark chocolate shavings

11 Before ganache sets, sprinkle shaved dark chocolate on top of the cake.

12 Let the ganache set before slicing and serving. Store frosted cake covered in the refrigerator up to 1 week.

Per Serving
Calories: 344 | Fat: 30g | Protein: 8g | Sodium: 189mg | Fiber: 8g | Carbohydrates: 32g | Net Carbohydrates: 8g | Sugar: 3g | Sugar Alcohol: 4g

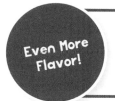

Even More Flavor!

A secret tip to deepen the flavor of this cake even more—coffee! Reduce the milk to ¹/₂ cup and add ¹/₄ cup of cooled espresso or double-strength coffee. It will enhance the natural flavor of the chocolate even more!

Texas Chocolate Sheet Cake

This is a minimal-effort cake and it comes together quick. And bonus: There's no need to wait for the cake to cool before frosting it.

CAKE

1 tablespoon coconut oil, for the pan

½ cup whole milk

1 teaspoon apple cider vinegar

12 tablespoons unsalted butter, slightly softened

⅔ cup granulated (or crystalized) allulose sweetener

4 large eggs

1 tablespoon pure vanilla extract

½ teaspoon liquid stevia

2 cups almond flour

⅓ cup unsweetened cocoa powder

¼ cup golden flaxseed meal

2 teaspoons baking powder

¾ teaspoon salt

½ teaspoon psyllium husk powder

¼ teaspoon instant espresso powder

⅛ teaspoon baking soda

FROSTING

8 tablespoons unsalted butter

⅓ cup whole milk

⅓ cup unsweetened cocoa powder

⅛ teaspoon salt

1¼ cups powdered allulose sweetener

1 teaspoon pure vanilla extract

1 *For the Cake:* Preheat oven to 350°F. Grease the sides of a half-sheet pan (18" × 13" × 1") with coconut oil and place a piece of parchment paper that's been trimmed to fit in the bottom.

2 To a large bowl, add milk and sprinkle on vinegar. Let it sit 3 minutes without moving the bowl or stirring it while milk curdles. Beat in butter, granulated allulose, eggs, vanilla, and stevia.

3 Beat in almond flour, cocoa powder, flaxseed meal, baking powder, salt, psyllium husk powder, espresso powder, and baking soda.

4 Transfer batter into the prepared pan and spread it out evenly all the way to the edges. Bake until a toothpick inserted in the center comes out clean, about 12–15 minutes.

5 *For the Frosting:* To a medium saucepan over medium heat, add butter, milk, cocoa powder, and salt, stirring occasionally. Bring to a boil and then let it boil vigorously for 1 minute, whisking occasionally. Remove from heat and whisk in powdered allulose and vanilla.

6 *To Frost the Cake:* While cake and frosting are both still hot, carefully pour frosting over cake and spread it out evenly with a rubber spatula.

7 Once it's frosted, let the cake sit at least 15 minutes before cutting and serving. This cake can be eaten hot or cold.

8 Store leftover cake covered at room temperature up to 2 days, or covered in the refrigerator up to 1 week.

Per Serving
Calories: 176 | Fat: 16g | Protein: 4g | Sodium: 149mg | Fiber: 2g | Carbohydrates: 17g | Net Carbohydrates: 2g | Sugar: 1g

Chocolate Hazelnut Bark

The last time we were in Paris, we fell in love with chocolate all over again. Deep, dark chocolate with toasted whole hazelnuts to be exact! The nutty crunch of hazelnut is the perfect way to offset the rich velvetiness of chocolate. We recommend enjoying this bark with a cup of espresso.

150 grams (about 2 bars) stevia-sweetened 70% cocoa dark chocolate, such as Lily's

½ cup whole hazelnuts, toasted

1 Line a large baking sheet with parchment paper.

2 In a microwave-safe bowl or double boiler, melt dark chocolate.

3 In a large bowl, stir together melted chocolate and whole hazelnuts.

4 Spread out mixture on the prepared baking sheet until it's about ¼" thick.

5 Let bark set and then break it into pieces. Store in an airtight container in the refrigerator up to 1 month.

Per Serving
Calories: 178 | Fat: 16g | Protein: 4g | Sodium: 0mg | Fiber: 8g | Carbohydrates: 14g | Net Carbohydrates: 2g | Sugar: 0g | Sugar Alcohol: 4g

Can You Make Bars Instead of Bark?

Yes! Use your favorite candy bar molds and pour in the chocolate mixture. Let it set, and then remove from the molds.

Cake Pops

The really fun part about this recipe (other than eating the Cake Pops) is that it's a cake smash! Crumble up the cake, mix it with butter, roll it into balls, coat it in chocolate, and revel in the fact that your Cake Pops are not only keto, but also as good as anything you'd get at a bakery.

¼ of a Basic Vanilla Cake, unfrosted (see recipe in this chapter)

½ cup Basic Buttercream, at room temperature (see recipe in this chapter)

5 ounces 90% cocoa dark chocolate

8 (4") lollipop sticks

1 Crumble Basic Vanilla Cake in a large bowl (you should get about 1¾ cups of crumbled cake).

2 Beat Basic Buttercream into crumbled cake until it comes together like a dough.

3 Scoop the mixture into eight balls (2 tablespoons each). Place balls on a parchment paper–lined tray and chill in the freezer 10 minutes.

4 In a microwave-safe bowl or double boiler, melt dark chocolate. Dip each cake ball in melted chocolate, letting excess drip off, and place them on a wax paper–lined tray. If there is any chocolate left over, drizzle it decoratively on top.

5 Place a lollipop stick in the center of each pop.

6 Let chocolate set before serving. Store in an airtight container in the refrigerator up to 2 weeks.

Per Serving
Calories: 235 | Fat: 21g | Protein: 4g | Sodium: 106mg | Fiber: 3g | Carbohydrates: 21g | Net Carbohydrates: 2g | Sugar: 2g

Make Them Birthday Cake Pops!

Celebrate the big day with your Funfetti-loving friends and family! And yes, you can find keto-friendly sprinkles. Our favorite is Good Dee's Sugar Free Sprinkles, which you can buy online.

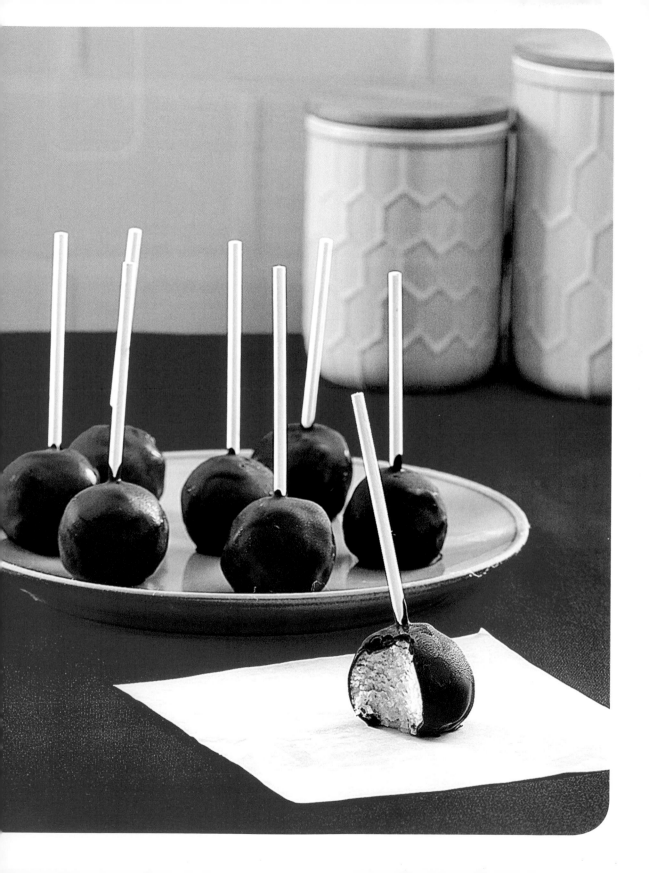

Tiramisu Parfait

You'll think you walked into a café in Rome with these Tiramisu Parfaits! The flavor of espresso pairs perfectly with a sweet vanilla mascarpone cream and vanilla cake. The best part is, these keep well up to 5 days in the refrigerator, so you can make them ahead of time.

8 ounces mascarpone cheese, at room temperature

½ cup heavy whipping cream

3 tablespoons powdered allulose sweetener

1 teaspoon pure vanilla extract

½ teaspoon vanilla bean paste

¼ of a Basic Vanilla Cake, unfrosted (see recipe in this chapter)

4 tablespoons espresso, cooled

1½ teaspoons unsweetened cocoa powder

1 In a large mixing bowl, beat together mascarpone, cream, powdered allulose, vanilla extract, and vanilla bean paste.

2 Let cake cool completely (this works best if you make the cake a day or two in advance and let it chill in the refrigerator so it dries out a little), and then cut it into small (about ¼") cubes.

3 Get out six (6-ounce) juice glasses. Add about 1½ tablespoons cubed cake to the bottom of each juice glass. Drizzle 1 teaspoon espresso on cake in each glass. Top each with about 1 tablespoon mascarpone mixture and smooth them out. Divide remaining cake between each glass, and drizzle 1 teaspoon espresso onto cake. Top with remaining mascarpone mixture. Smooth out the tops.

4 Sprinkle ¼ teaspoon cocoa powder on top of each parfait.

5 Cover and chill at least 1 hour before serving.

Per Serving
Calories: 325 | Fat: 29g | Protein: 6g | Sodium: 153mg | Fiber: 1g | Carbohydrates: 18g | Net Carbohydrates: 7g | Sugar: 3g

Do You Need to Use Espresso?

Instead of espresso, you can use double-strength coffee in this recipe.

Chocolate Coconut Bites

For the chocolate coconut candy bar lover in all of us, we had to share our Chocolate Coconut Bites! Use them as fat bombs or as dessert. Or a snack. Or just anytime a chocolate craving hits.

¾ cup heavy whipping cream

3 tablespoons unsalted butter

1½ tablespoons Swerve Confectioners

10 drops liquid stevia

¹⁄₁₆ teaspoon salt

1 teaspoon pure vanilla extract

1 cup shredded unsweetened coconut

5 ounces stevia-sweetened dark chocolate

1 To a medium saucepan over medium heat, add cream, butter, Swerve Confectioners, stevia, and salt. Bring mixture to a boil, and then let it continue boiling until it's thick and glossy, about 4–5 minutes, whisking frequently. It should be reduced to about ½–⅔ cup.

2 Remove from heat, whisk in vanilla, and stir in coconut. Cool to room temperature.

3 Place a piece of plastic wrap directly on top of the coconut mixture. Put mixture in the freezer until firm enough to shape into balls when squeezed, about 10 minutes.

4 Divide mixture into ten equal parts and shape each into a ball, squeezing gently so they hold their shape. Freeze for 5–10 minutes.

5 In a microwave-safe bowl or double boiler, melt dark chocolate. Dip each coconut ball into chocolate, and then place it on a tray lined with wax paper or parchment paper. Let the chocolate set before serving.

6 Serve or store in an airtight container in the refrigerator up to 2 weeks.

Per Serving (Serving size: 1 piece)
Calories: 195 | Fat: 19g | Protein: 2g | Sodium: 7mg | Fiber: 6g | Carbohydrates: 13g | Net Carbohydrates: 3g | Sugar: 1g | Sugar Alcohol: 4g

Chocolate-Covered Cherries

Was anyone else a fan of the classic candy called cherry cordials? They're the inspiration for these Chocolate-Covered Cherries, but these aren't sickly sweet and they won't make you sugar crash. Eat these as is like bonbons or use them to top your favorite keto ice cream sundae.

100 grams (about 1¼ bars) 90% cocoa dark chocolate, chopped or broken into pieces

20 frozen pitted sweet cherries

1 In a microwave-safe bowl or double boiler, melt dark chocolate.

2 Dip a frozen cherry into the chocolate, remove it with a fork, and let excess chocolate run off. Place cherry on a parchment paper–lined tray. Continue until all the cherries are dipped.

3 Serve, or place on a paper towel–lined plate and store in the refrigerator up to 2 hours.

Per Serving (Serving size: 2 pieces)
Calories: 67 | Fat: 6g | Protein: 1g | Sodium: 2mg | Fiber: 2g | Carbohydrates: 5g | Net Carbohydrates: 3g | Sugar: 2g

Can You Make These Ahead of Time?

We don't recommend making these more than 2 hours in advance because the chocolate can start to condense.

CHAPTER 8

Ice Cream Shop

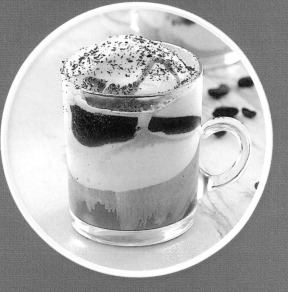

Vanilla Ice Cream

This ice cream is the perfect balance between rich and creamy and light and airy. Egg yolks help thicken it up and give it an old-fashioned frozen custard flavor. A double dose of vanilla in the form of vanilla extract and vanilla bean paste provides deep flavor with the perfect amount of sweetness.

5 large egg yolks

3 cups heavy whipping cream, divided

¼ cup powdered allulose sweetener

3 tablespoons pure MCT oil

1 tablespoon vodka

1 tablespoon pure vanilla extract

½ tablespoon vanilla bean paste

⅛ teaspoon liquid stevia

1/16 teaspoon salt

Can You Skip the MCT Oil and Vodka?

These two ingredients help yield the best texture for this ice cream, so we don't suggest skipping them. These ingredients help make sure this ice cream doesn't freeze into a solid block and still has smooth, creamy texture even after a couple months. Straight out of the freezer, we recommend letting this ice cream sit at room temperature for 15 minutes before scooping, or you can microwave it for 15-second increments.

1 Place egg yolks in a large bowl.

2 In a medium saucepan, add 2 cups cream and powdered allulose. Bring to a simmer over medium heat.

3 Once simmering, slowly drizzle hot cream into egg yolks while whisking until cream is fully incorporated.

4 Return cream and yolk mixture to the saucepan. Bring to a simmer over medium heat, whisking continuously.

5 Remove from heat and whisk in MCT oil, vodka, vanilla extract, vanilla bean paste, stevia, and salt.

6 Strain through a fine-mesh sieve, then cool to room temperature. Place a piece of plastic wrap directly on top of custard mixture. Refrigerate until chilled, about 4 hours.

7 In a large bowl, beat remaining 1 cup cream with a stand mixer or a handheld electric mixer until it reaches medium peaks.

8 Whisk ¼ of whipped cream into custard mixture, and then fold in remaining ¾ whipped cream ¼ at a time. Try not to fully deflate whipped cream.

9 Pour ice cream into a freezer-safe container, cover container, and freeze 1 hour. Stir ice cream, and then re-cover container and freeze 1 hour.

10 Stir ice cream again, re-cover container, and then freeze until solid. Serve.

11 Store any leftover ice cream in a covered container in the freezer up to 6 months.

Per Serving (Serving size: 1/3 cup)
Calories: 247 | Fat: 24g | Protein: 2g | Sodium: 35mg | Fiber: 0g | Carbohydrates: 5g | Net Carbohydrates: 2g | Sugar: 2g

Hot Fudge

Rich, gooey, decadent, and deeply chocolatey, this Hot Fudge delivers in every way. Drizzle it on any keto ice cream you dish up or use it to make something a little more special, like our Kitchen Sink Ice Cream Sundae or Chocolate Overload Milkshake (see recipes in this chapter).

1½ cups heavy whipping cream

6 tablespoons unsalted butter

½ cup powdered allulose sweetener

3 tablespoons unsweetened cocoa powder

2 tablespoons brewed strong coffee

20 drops liquid stevia

1/16 teaspoon salt

1 teaspoon pure vanilla extract

2 ounces 90% cocoa dark chocolate, chopped

1 To a medium saucepan, add cream, butter, powdered allulose, cocoa powder, coffee, stevia, and salt.

2 Bring to a boil, and then cook until thickened and it looks like molten lava, about 5–6 minutes. It will thicken more as it cools, so don't overcook it.

3 Remove from heat and stir in vanilla and then dark chocolate. Serve warm.

4 Let any leftover Hot Fudge cool to room temperature, and then put it in an airtight container and store in the refrigerator up to 2 weeks.

Per Serving (Serving size: 2 tablespoons)
Calories: 184 | Fat: 19g | Protein: 1g | Sodium: 25mg | Fiber: 1g | Carbohydrates: 9g | Net Carbohydrates: 2g | Sugar: 1g

How to Reheat Leftover Hot Fudge

This Hot Fudge reheats well in the microwave in 15-second increments (stirring after each increment) or in a double boiler. Note that it will thicken after it's refrigerated, but it will thin out to hot fudge consistency after reheating.

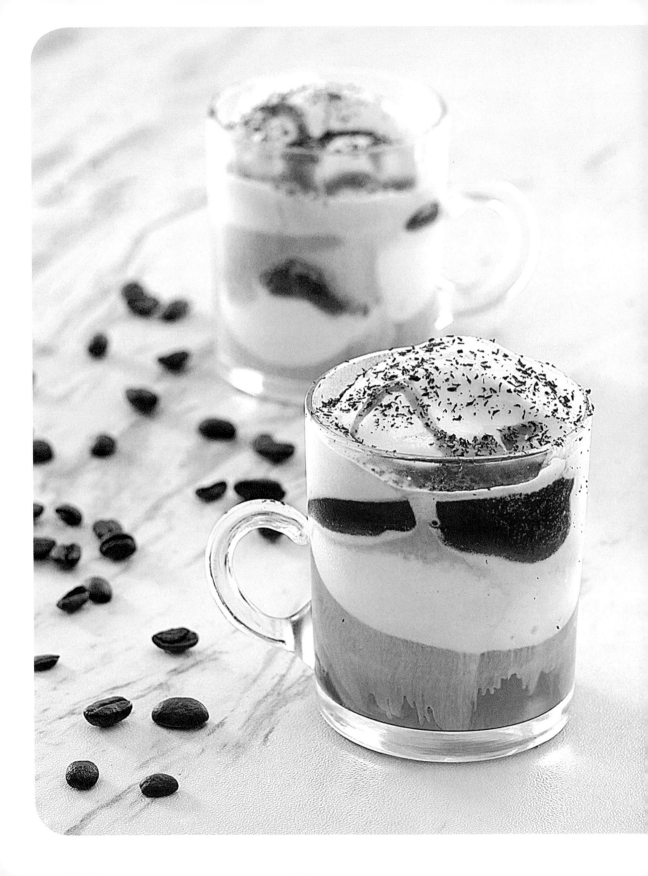

Loaded Affogato

Affogato (meaning "drowned") is an Italian treat that combines vanilla ice cream or gelato with espresso. We take it to the next level with a drizzle of Caramel Sauce and a sprinkle of super dark chocolate shavings.

¼ cup Vanilla Ice Cream (see recipe in this chapter)

1 shot hot espresso

1 tablespoon Caramel Sauce, warm (see recipe in this chapter)

1 teaspoon 90% dark chocolate shavings, for garnish

Add ice cream to a small glass. Pour on espresso. Drizzle on Caramel Sauce. Top with dark chocolate shavings. Serve.

Per Serving
Calories: 303 | Fat: 28g | Protein: 2g | Sodium: 51mg | Fiber: 0g | Carbohydrates: 12g | Net Carbohydrates: 5g | Sugar: 4g

Caramel Sauce

Caramel Sauce is the antithesis to Hot Fudge, and every good ice cream shop offers both. You'll be surprised by how much this version reminds you of regular caramel! It's sweet with subtle notes of burnt sugar and vanilla and has a beautiful golden color.

4 tablespoons unsalted butter

¼ cup granulated (or crystallized) allulose sweetener

¾ cup heavy whipping cream

½ teaspoon blackstrap molasses

½ teaspoon pure vanilla extract

¼ teaspoon cream of tartar

⅛ teaspoon liquid stevia

1/16 teaspoon salt

1 In a medium saucepan over medium heat, add butter and allulose. Bring to a boil, whisking occasionally. Let it boil until it turns a light golden brown, about 2 minutes, whisking frequently. Be careful not to scorch it.

2 Whisk in cream, molasses, vanilla, cream of tartar, stevia, and salt. Bring mixture back to a boil, and then let it boil until it's thickened and looks like molten lava, about 3–4 minutes, whisking occasionally. Don't overcook it; it will thicken more as it cools.

3 Cool slightly and then serve.

4 Let any leftover Caramel Sauce cool to room temperature, and then put it in an airtight container and store in the refrigerator up to 2 weeks.

Per Serving (Serving size: 2 tablespoons)
Calories: 175 | Fat: 18g | Protein: 1g | Sodium: 36mg | Fiber: 0g | Carbohydrates: 9g | Net Carbohydrates: 1g | Sugar: 1g

What Is the Cream of Tartar For?

Don't skip out on the cream of tartar here! It helps prevent crystallization so your Caramel Sauce is silky smooth.

Kitchen Sink Ice Cream Sundae

This mash-up of a bunch of different desserts is the best excuse we know to make a bunch of different recipes from this cookbook. That way you can figure out which ones are your favorite and then have a little dessert party and make this sundae! Don't let the (relatively) small serving size surprise you. Keto desserts are low in carbs but not low in calories, and they're very filling.

1 cup Vanilla Ice Cream (see recipe in this chapter)

1 Brownie Bite, cut in 4 pieces (see Chapter 7)

1 slice Basic Vanilla Cake, crumbled slightly (see Chapter 7)

2 tablespoons Hot Fudge, warm (see recipe in this chapter)

2 tablespoons Caramel Sauce, warm (see recipe in this chapter)

2 Chocolate Coconut Bites, chopped (see Chapter 7)

4 Chocolate-Covered Cherries (see Chapter 7)

1 To serve sharing style, add all ingredients to a large, shallow bowl. Serve.

2 To serve individual style, divide all ingredients between four small bowls. Serve.

Per Serving
Calories: 534 | Fat: 50g | Protein: 7g | Sodium: 121mg | Fiber: 6g | Carbohydrates: 26g | Net Carbohydrates: 7g | Sugar: 4g | Sugar Alcohol: 2g

Ice Cream Sundae Waffle

Is it breakfast? Is it dessert? Does it matter?! This decadent dish is sure to make your sweet tooth swoon.

SWEET WAFFLES

4 tablespoons unsalted butter, melted and cooled slightly

6 ounces cream cheese, softened

4 large eggs

1 tablespoon pure vanilla extract

¾ cup almond flour

¼ cup granulated (or crystalized) allulose sweetener

1 teaspoon psyllium husk powder

1 teaspoon baking powder

¼ teaspoon salt

1 cup pre-shredded low-moisture part-skim mozzarella cheese

Coconut oil spray

OTHER

1 cup Vanilla Ice Cream (see recipe in this chapter)

4 tablespoons Hot Fudge (see recipe in this chapter)

2 tablespoons Caramel Sauce (see recipe in this chapter)

4 fresh cherries

1 *For the Sweet Waffles:* In a large bowl, whisk together butter, cream cheese, eggs, and vanilla. Whisk in almond flour, allulose, psyllium husk powder, baking powder, and salt until combined. Stir in mozzarella. Let batter rest 2 minutes to thicken.

2 Plug in a waffle iron. Once heated, spray the inside with coconut oil .

3 Pour ¼ of batter into the heated waffle iron and cook until waffle starts to steam, about 2–3 minutes. Carefully remove cooked waffle and cook remaining batter the same way.

4 *To Make the Waffle Sundaes:* Place the four waffles on four plates. Top each with ¼ cup Vanilla Ice Cream, 1 tablespoon Hot Fudge, ½ tablespoon Caramel Sauce, and 1 cherry. Serve.

Per Serving
Calories: 887 | Fat: 76g | Protein: 22g | Sodium: 718mg | Fiber: 3g | Carbohydrates: 32g | Net Carbohydrates: 9g | Sugar: 6g

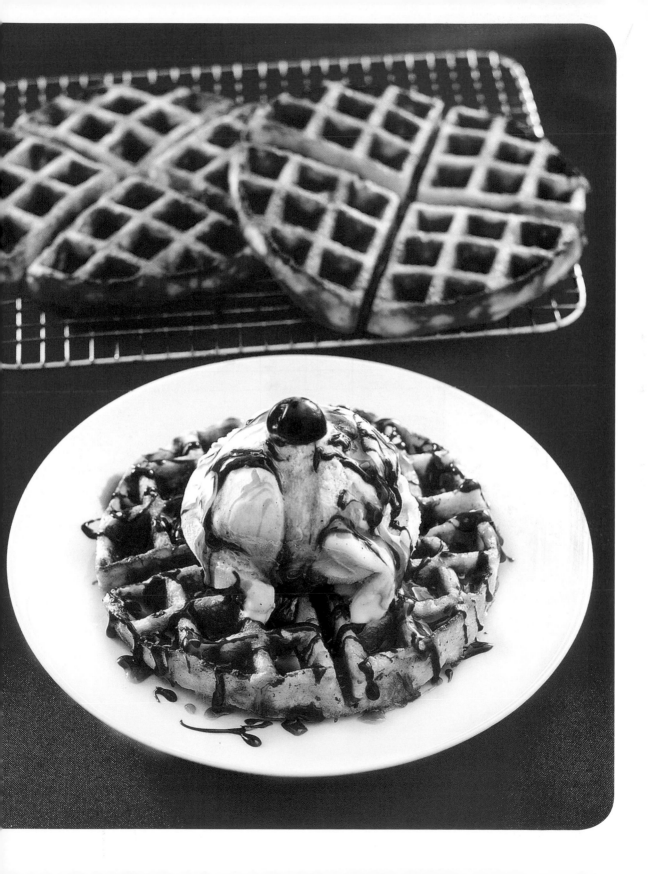

Cookie Dough Ice Cream Sundae

Cookie dough plus vanilla ice cream is a match made in heaven, and our Hot Fudge only makes it better. Feel free to make a double or triple batch of this and freeze it in individual portions so they're ready for when a craving hits.

¼ cup Edible Cookie Dough (see Chapter 7)

⅔ cup Vanilla Ice Cream (see recipe in this chapter)

3 tablespoons Hot Fudge, warm (see recipe in this chapter)

1 Line a plate with a piece of wax paper. Scoop cookie dough into ½-tablespoon balls and place them on the prepared plate so they're not touching. Freeze to firm them slightly, about 10 minutes.

2 Add ice cream to two small bowls. Top with cookie dough balls. Drizzle on Hot Fudge. Serve.

Per Serving
Calories: 497 | Fat: 48g | Protein: 5g | Sodium: 135mg | Fiber: 4g | Carbohydrates: 21g | Net Carbohydrates: 6g | Sugar: 3g

Ultimate "Breakfast" Milkshake

Okay, so this milkshake probably isn't breakfast. But it does have a few different breakfast components! Instead of drizzling keto maple-flavored syrup on top, you can add 2 tablespoons of fresh blueberries for a pop of fresh flavor.

CANDIED BACON

Avocado oil spray

2 teaspoons keto brown sugar

2 slices beef bacon

VANILLA MILKSHAKE

1/3 cup Vanilla Ice Cream (see recipe in this chapter)

1/2 cup ice cubes

1/2 cup plain, unsweetened almond milk

1/2 teaspoon vanilla bean paste

7 drops liquid stevia

OTHER

1/2 of a Sweet Waffle (see Ice Cream Sundae Waffle recipe in this chapter)

2 teaspoons keto maple-flavored syrup

1 *For the Candied Bacon:* Preheat oven to 375°F. Line a large baking sheet with foil and then place a wire rack on top. Spray the rack with avocado oil.

2 Massage brown sugar into bacon slices. Lay bacon slices flat on the wire rack. Bake until the sugar is melted and the bacon is golden, about 18–25 minutes, and then cool to room temperature. The bacon will crisp more as it cools.

3 *For the Vanilla Milkshake:* Add all ingredients to a blender and purée until smooth, tamping down as necessary.

4 *To Assemble and Serve:* Pour milkshake into two glasses.

5 Cut the Sweet Waffle in half. Tuck one half of the waffle into each milkshake. Drizzle maple-flavored syrup on top. Serve immediately.

Per Serving
Calories: 381 | Fat: 33g | Protein: 11g | Sodium: 532mg | Fiber: 3g | Carbohydrates: 15g | Net Carbohydrates: 4g | Sugar: 2g | Sugar Alcohol: 3g

Make a Big Batch of Candied Bacon (You Won't Regret It)

This bacon is so delicious and it doesn't really take much more effort to make a bigger batch, so go ahead and do it! For 8 slices of beef bacon, use 8 teaspoons of keto brown sugar. Each serving is two slices, and you'll get about four servings from this amount.

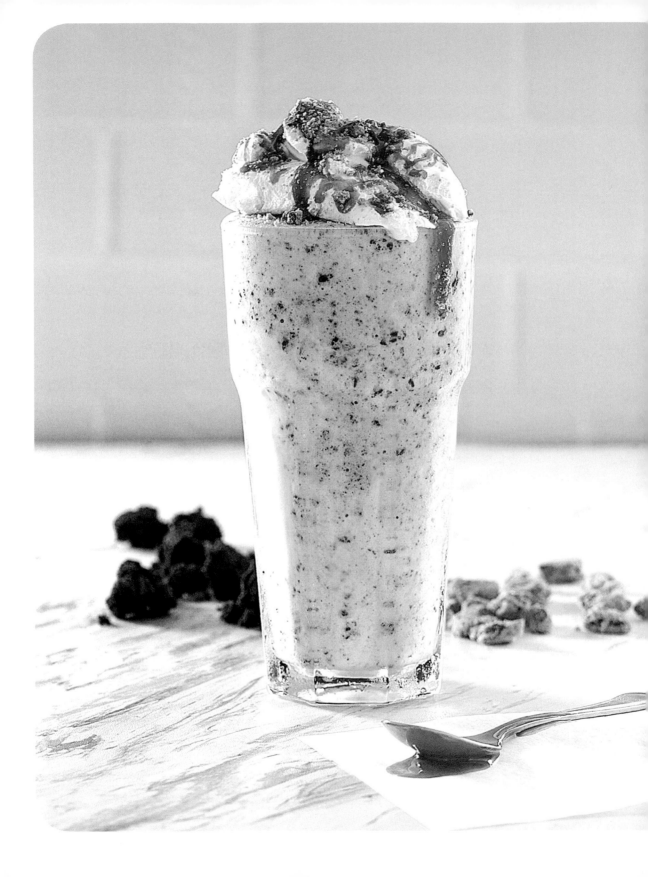

Cookies and Cream Milkshake

Think of this milkshake flavor as the love child of cookie dough ice cream and cookies and cream ice cream. We live in a world where you don't have to choose just one favorite!

VANILLA MILKSHAKE

1/3 cup Vanilla Ice Cream (see recipe in this chapter)

1/2 cup ice cubes

1/2 cup plain, unsweetened almond milk

1/2 teaspoon vanilla bean paste

7 drops liquid stevia

OTHER

2 Chocolate Chip Cookies (see Chapter 7)

1/2 Brownie Bite (see Chapter 7)

2 tablespoons whipped cream, whipped to soft peaks

2 tablespoons Caramel Sauce (see recipe in this chapter)

1 *For the Vanilla Milkshake:* Add all ingredients to a blender and purée until smooth, tamping down as necessary.

2 Add 1 Chocolate Chip Cookie and the 1/2 Brownie Bite and pulse a couple times.

3 *To Assemble and Serve:* Pour milkshake into two glasses.

4 Top each milkshake with whipped cream, crumble remaining Chocolate Chip Cookie on top, and drizzle on Caramel Sauce. Serve immediately.

Per Serving
Calories: 376 | Fat: 35g | Protein: 5g | Sodium: 121mg | Fiber: 3g | Carbohydrates: 19g | Net Carbohydrates: 6g | Sugar: 3g | Sugar Alcohol: 4g

Chocolate Overload Milkshake

Is there actually such a thing as chocolate overload? Not to us! This shake is rich, creamy, and deeply chocolatey with bits of brownie bites. Our gooey Hot Fudge goes on top, and whipped cream and chocolate chips complete the indulgence.

CHOCOLATE MILKSHAKE

⅓ cup Vanilla Ice Cream (see recipe in this chapter)

½ cup ice cubes

½ cup plain, unsweetened almond milk

2 tablespoons unsweetened cocoa powder

½ teaspoon vanilla bean paste

12 drops liquid stevia

OTHER

1 Brownie Bite (see Chapter 7)

2 tablespoons Hot Fudge, warm (see recipe in this chapter)

2 tablespoons whipped cream, whipped to soft peaks

1 teaspoon stevia-sweetened mini chocolate chips

1 *For the Chocolate Milkshake:* Add all ingredients to a blender and purée until smooth, tamping down as necessary.

2 Add the Brownie Bite and pulse a couple times.

3 *To Assemble and Serve:* Pour milkshake into two glasses.

4 Drizzle on Hot Fudge, and dollop whipped cream on top of each glass. Top with chocolate chips. Serve immediately.

Per Serving
Calories: 396 | Fat: 37g | Protein: 6g | Sodium: 103mg | Fiber: 7g | Carbohydrates: 24g | Net Carbohydrates: 7g | Sugar: 3g | Sugar Alcohol: 2g

Your Not-So-Basic Vanilla Shake

Have you heard of the freakshake craze? Freakshakes are over-the-top decadent milkshakes that can be topped with cake slices, blended with cookies, stacked high with doughnuts, and so on. Of course, they're normally loaded with calories and sugar, but our keto rendition keeps the carbs at a minimum while still delivering big on the wow factor.

VANILLA MILKSHAKE

⅓ cup Vanilla Ice Cream (see recipe in this chapter)

½ cup ice cubes

½ cup plain, unsweetened almond milk

½ teaspoon vanilla bean paste

7 drops liquid stevia

OTHER

1 slice Basic Vanilla Cake frosted with Basic Buttercream (see Chapter 7)

1 teaspoon keto rainbow sprinkles

2 fresh cherries

1 *For the Vanilla Milkshake:* Add all ingredients to a blender and purée until smooth, tamping down as necessary.

2 *To Assemble and Serve:* Pour milkshake into two glasses.

3 Cut slice of cake in half. Coarsely crumble half of it and stir it into milkshakes. Balance a piece of the other half of cake slice on top of each glass. Top each with ½ teaspoon sprinkles and 1 cherry. Serve immediately.

Per Serving
Calories: 312 | Fat: 28g | Protein: 5g | Sodium: 202mg | Fiber: 2g | Carbohydrates: 26g | Net Carbohydrates: 5g | Sugar: 3g | Sugar Alcohol: 1g

You Just Want a Regular Vanilla Milkshake?

You've found your new go-to recipe! Make the Vanilla Milkshake part of this recipe (it makes 1 serving) and top it with a little whipped cream.

CHAPTER 9

Happy Hour Drinks & Bar Bites

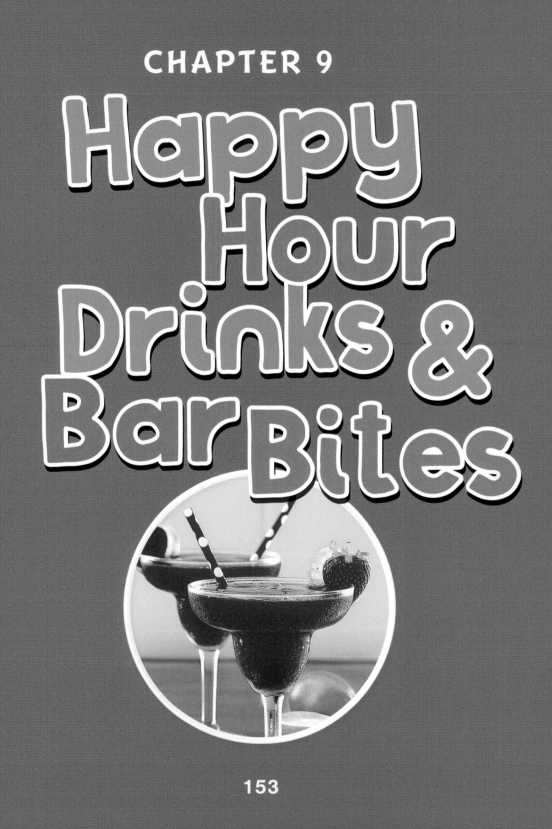

Piña Colada

White sandy beaches, blue skies, turquoise water. Mix up a Piña Colada and feel like you're transported to paradise! Don't forget the little umbrella and a colorful straw.

6 ounces light rum
¾ teaspoon pineapple extract
¼ teaspoon coconut extract
3 ounces canned unsweetened full-fat coconut milk
Ice, as needed

1 Add rum, pineapple extract, coconut extract, and coconut milk to a mixer glass and stir.

2 Pour the drink into two poco grande glasses, each filled with a handful of ice. Serve.

Per Serving
Calories: 285 | Fat: 9g | Protein: 1g | Sodium: 6mg | Fiber: 0g | Carbohydrates: 1g | Net Carbohydrates: 1g | Sugar: 0g

Make This One Frozen!

We love a good frozen Piña Colada on a hot day! To serve this drink frozen, just blend up everything in a blender. If desired, add keto sweetener (such as liquid stevia) to taste.

White Russian

To nix the carbs, instead of using the traditional Kahlúa for this cocktail, we use espresso. Alternatively, you can use double-strength regular coffee that's cooled. Feel free to make it decaf if you're enjoying this cocktail in the evening!

Ice, as needed
6 ounces vodka
2 ounces cooled espresso
2 ounces heavy whipping cream

Fill two old fashioned glasses with ice. Into each, pour 3 ounces vodka and 1 ounce cooled espresso. Pour 1 ounce cream into each, and then stir. Serve.

Per Serving
Calories: 296 | Fat: 10g | Protein: 1g | Sodium: 14mg | Fiber: 0g | Carbohydrates: 1g | Net Carbohydrates: 1g | Sugar: 1g

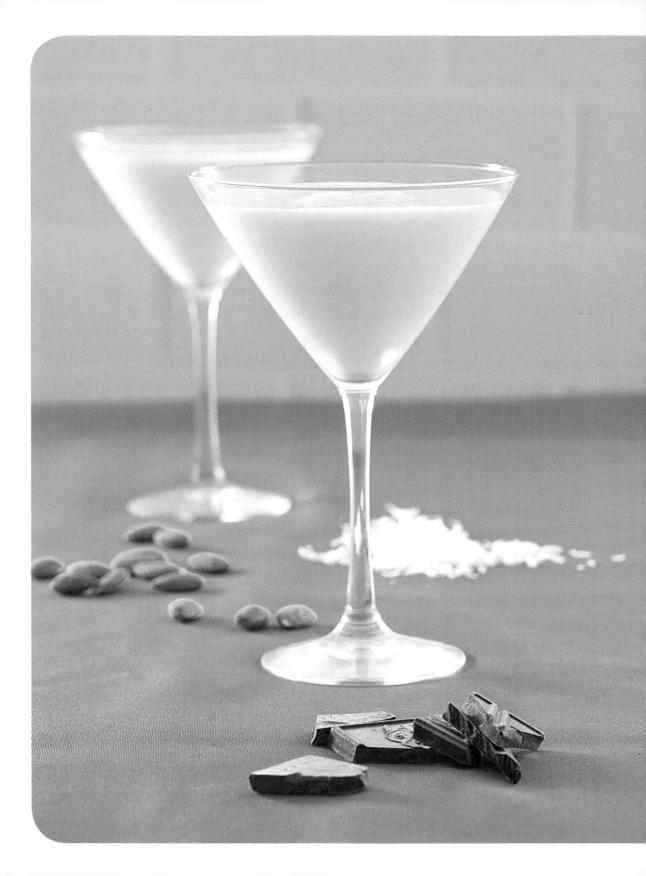

Chocolate Almond Coconut Martinis

If you like Almond Joy candy bars, this will be your favorite new cocktail! Vodka has no carbs, so we went with that and used a variety of extracts to come up with the same flavor profile. Feel free to tweak the amount of each extract to suit your tastes.

6 ounces vodka
¼ teaspoon coconut extract
¼ teaspoon chocolate extract
¼ teaspoon almond extract
2 ounces heavy whipping cream
Ice, as needed

1 Add vodka, coconut extract, chocolate extract, almond extract, and cream to a shaker bottle filled with ice and shake.

2 Strain into two martini glasses. Serve.

Per Serving
Calories: 298 | Fat: 10g | Protein: 1g | Sodium: 11mg | Fiber: 0g | Carbohydrates: 1g | Net Carbohydrates: 1g | Sugar: 1g

Funky Monkey Martini

Peanut butter, banana, and chocolate combine in this fun and whimsical drink. If you want, you can play with the alcohol and use light rum instead of vodka. A coconut rim is the perfect finishing touch!

1 tablespoon powdered allulose sweetener

½ tablespoon water

1 tablespoon unsweetened shredded coconut

Ice, as needed

6 ounces vodka

½ teaspoon peanut butter extract

¼ teaspoon banana extract

¼ teaspoon chocolate extract

2 ounces heavy whipping cream

7 drops liquid stevia

1 Put powdered allulose and water in a small saucepan over medium heat. Stir until allulose is dissolved, and then remove from heat. Cool, and then transfer to a shallow bowl (it will be a very small amount).

2 Put coconut in a separate shallow bowl.

3 Dip rims of two martini glasses in dissolved allulose liquid and then in coconut.

4 To a shaker bottle filled with ice, add vodka, peanut butter extract, banana extract, chocolate extract, cream, and stevia and shake.

5 Strain the drink into the prepared glasses. Serve.

Per Serving
Calories: 316 | Fat: 11g | Protein: 1g | Sodium: 11mg | Fiber: 1g | Carbohydrates: 6g | Net Carbohydrates: 1g | Sugar: 1g

Classic Margs

Because if there aren't margaritas, is it really a party?! We thought you'd agree, and so we had to include a recipe here. Pair these with Chips and Queso (see Chapter 6) and maybe some homemade guacamole and let the good times roll (but don't forget, please drink responsibly!).

½ tablespoon coarse kosher salt

1 fresh lime wedge

5 ounces silver tequila

2 ounces fresh lime juice

2 tablespoons powdered allulose sweetener

1 teaspoon orange extract

4 cups ice cubes

1 Spread salt out on a small shallow plate. Run lime wedge around the rim of two margarita glasses. Immediately dip each in coarse salt.

2 To a blender, add tequila, lime juice, powdered allulose, orange extract, and ice cubes. Pulse a few times to break up the ice, and then process until the mixture is slushy.

3 Pour into the prepared glasses and serve immediately.

Per Serving
Calories: 176 | Fat: 0g | Protein: 0g | Sodium: 1,441mg | Fiber: 0g | Carbohydrates: 12g | Net Carbohydrates: 3g | Sugar: 1g

Strawberry Margs Are My Favorite, Though!

If you'd prefer a strawberry marg, just add 1 cup frozen strawberries and reduce the ice cubes to 3 cups!

Strawberry Daiquiris

Fun, fruity, and classic, this Strawberry Daiquiri hits all the right notes. Frozen strawberries are the key to this drink. They add thickness and flavor without watering down the drink. This cocktail is also delicious with frozen red raspberries instead of strawberries!

6 ounces light rum
1 cup frozen strawberries
1½ tablespoons powdered allulose sweetener
1 tablespoon fresh lime juice
½ cup ice cubes
2 fresh strawberries, for garnish
2 slices fresh lime, for garnish

1 Add rum, frozen strawberries, powdered allulose, lime juice, and ice cubes to a blender and pulse a few times to break up the strawberries. Purée until smooth.

2 Pour into two daiquiri glasses and garnish each with 1 strawberry and 1 lime slice. Serve.

Per Serving
Calories: 227 | Fat: 0g | Protein: 0g | Sodium: 1mg | Fiber: 2g | Carbohydrates: 15g | Net Carbohydrates: 6g | Sugar: 4g

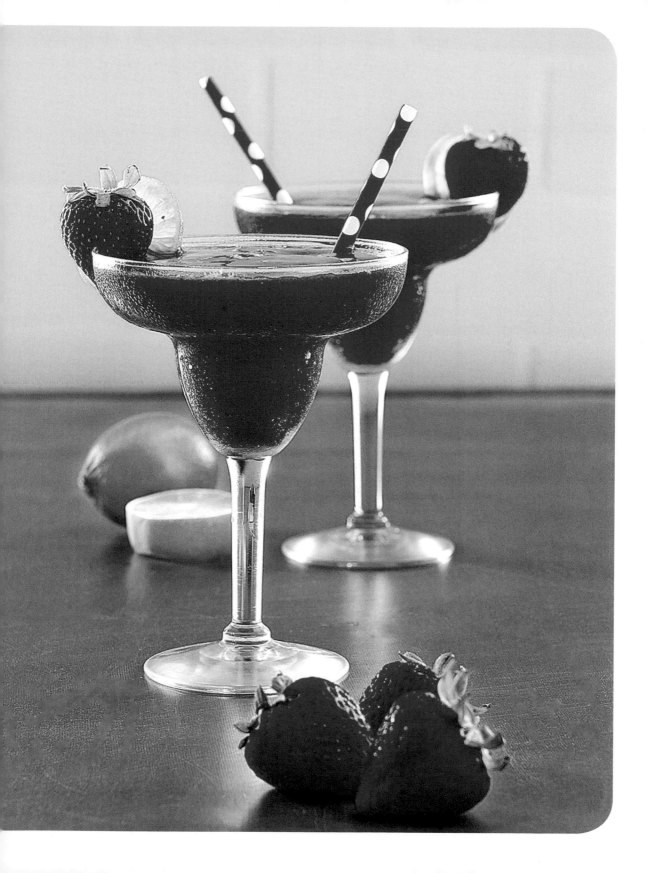

Herbed Almonds

Few things are better than taking an hour in the afternoon to enjoy a beverage and something to munch on. Herbed Almonds are the perfect choice. They're savory and fragrant and surprisingly addictive!

2 cups raw almonds

1 tablespoon extra-virgin olive oil

1 tablespoon minced fresh rosemary

½ tablespoon minced fresh thyme

½ teaspoon garlic powder

½ teaspoon salt

¼ teaspoon ground black pepper

1 Preheat oven to 350°F. Line a large baking sheet with parchment paper or a Silpat liner.

2 Toss together all ingredients and spread out on the prepared baking sheet.

3 Roast 5 minutes, and then carefully toss almonds. Return to oven and roast until almonds are golden and fragrant, about 5–10 minutes more.

4 Cool to room temperature, and then store in an airtight container at room temperature up to 1 month.

Per Serving
Calories: 176 | Fat: 16g | Protein: 6g | Sodium: 145mg | Fiber: 3g | Carbohydrates: 6g | Net Carbohydrates: 3g | Sugar: 1g

Give These Almonds a Kick

If you like it spicy, add ¼–½ teaspoon cayenne pepper along with the other spices.

Marinated Olives

Olives are an OG keto snack from way back. And they're a great thing to pair with a glass of dry red wine for happy hour at home! We recommend letting the olives marinate in this mixture for at least 2 hours before serving. For a nice variation in color and flavor, we like to use a mix of good-quality olives.

2 cups unpitted mixed olives, such as Kalamata, Cerignola, and Castelvetrano

3 medium cloves garlic, peeled and thinly sliced

2 tablespoons chopped fresh rosemary

½ teaspoon peppercorns

¼ teaspoon crushed red pepper flakes

2 (1") pieces fresh lemon peel

3 tablespoons extra-virgin olive oil

2 tablespoons white wine vinegar

1 Add all ingredients to a large bowl and stir to combine.

2 Cover and refrigerate at least 2 hours before serving.

3 Store covered in the refrigerator up to 2 weeks.

Per Serving
Calories: 61 | Fat: 7g | Protein: 0g | Sodium: 372mg | Fiber: 1g | Carbohydrates: 1g | Net Carbohydrates: 0g | Sugar: 0g

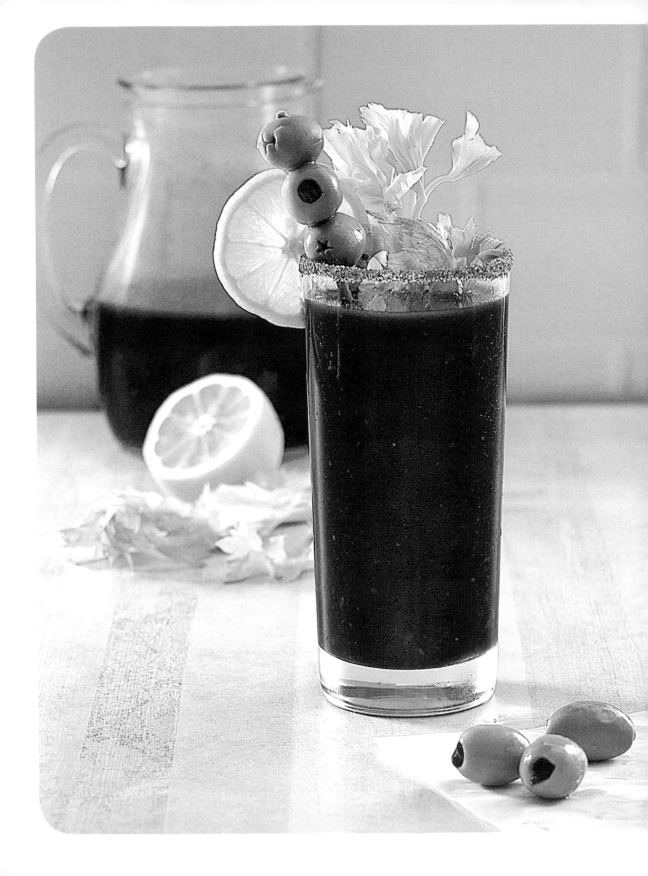

Bloody Marys

Savory, zippy, and slightly tangy with a little punch of heat, this Bloody Mary has a well-balanced flavor profile. If you like your Bloody Marys on the spicy side, Faith's grandmother recommends adding 1 ounce of pickled jalapeño juice (the juice that pickled jalapeños are in) and garnishing with a pickled jalapeño!

¾ teaspoon celery salt

1 fresh lemon wedge

¾ cup ice cubes

4 ounces no-sugar-added tomato juice

2 ounces vodka

½ tablespoon fresh lemon juice

1 teaspoon hot sauce

½ teaspoon Worcestershire sauce

¼ teaspoon horseradish

1/16 teaspoon ground black pepper, plus more for garnish if desired

1/16 teaspoon garlic powder

1/16 teaspoon smoked paprika

2 drops liquid stevia

3 green olives, skewered on a toothpick, for garnish

1 medium stalk celery, preferably with leaves, for garnish

1 lemon wheel, for garnish

1 Spread celery salt on a small shallow plate. Run lemon wedge around rim of a highball glass. Immediately dip it in the celery salt to coat the rim. Add ice cubes to the glass.

2 To a pitcher, add tomato juice, vodka, lemon juice, hot sauce, Worcestershire sauce, horseradish, black pepper, garlic powder, paprika, and stevia and stir well. Or to get it really well blended, process it in a blender.

3 Pour tomato juice mixture into the prepared glass. Garnish with olive skewer, celery stalk, and lemon wheel. Add a pinch of black pepper on top if desired. Serve immediately.

Per Serving
Calories: 178 | Fat: 1g | Protein: 1g | Sodium: 1,496mg | Fiber: 2g | Carbohydrates: 8g | Net Carbohydrates: 6g | Sugar: 4g

Goat Cheese–Stuffed Peppers

When it comes to elegant appetizers that are as customizable as they are delicious, Goat Cheese–Stuffed Peppers are a winner! If goat cheese isn't your thing, swap it out for cream cheese, ricotta cheese, cottage cheese, or farmer's cheese, and use any fresh herbs you like. These little bites are great served hot or cold.

1 (8-ounce) goat cheese log, at room temperature

2 ounces shredded sharp white Cheddar cheese

1 medium clove garlic, peeled and crushed

4 teaspoons minced fresh scallions, divided

⅛ teaspoon salt

⅛ teaspoon ground black pepper

12 mini bell peppers, halved lengthwise and seeded

1 In a large bowl, use a stand mixer or a handheld electric mixer to beat goat cheese until smooth and creamy. Beat in Cheddar, garlic, 2 teaspoons scallions, salt, and black pepper.

2 Divide goat cheese mixture between mini bell pepper halves. Sprinkle remaining 2 teaspoons scallions on top.

3 Serve, or cover and refrigerate up to one day before serving.

Per Serving
Calories: 290 | Fat: 20g | Protein: 17g | Sodium: 399mg | Fiber: 1g | Carbohydrates: 6g | Net Carbohydrates: 5g | Sugar: 3g

Some Like It Hot!

To serve this as a hot appetizer, brush a baking sheet with avocado oil. Once the peppers are stuffed but before you sprinkle the scallions on top, arrange the peppers on the baking sheet. Broil them until the cheese is melted and starting to turn golden in spots (stay with it; this can happen fast under the broiler). Sprinkle the scallions on top and serve warm. And if by "hot" you mean spicy hot, add 1 minced jalapeño or ¼ teaspoon ground cayenne pepper to the goat cheese mixture.

Long Island Iced Tea

Although this classic cocktail looks like a tall glass of iced tea (and a lot of people claim it tastes like iced tea too!), there's actually no tea in it. Use your favorite brand of stevia-sweetened cola to make it.

1 ounce vodka

1 ounce light rum

1 ounce silver tequila

1 ounce gin

1 ounce fresh lemon juice

3 drops orange extract

7 drops liquid stevia

4 ounces stevia-sweetened cola

1 cup ice cubes

2 lemon wedges, for garnish

1 To a pitcher, add vodka, rum, tequila, gin, lemon juice, orange extract, and stevia and stir to combine.

2 Divide vodka mixture between two collins glasses. Add 2 ounces cola to each glass and gently stir to combine.

3 Add $\frac{1}{2}$ cup ice to each glass, garnish each with a lemon wedge, and serve immediately.

Per Serving
Calories: 135 | Fat: 0g | Protein: 0g | Sodium: 0mg | Fiber: 0g | Carbohydrates: 1g | Net Carbohydrates: 1g | Sugar: 0g

Whiskey Sours

This drink is a beautiful balance of sweet/tart flavor that's accentuated by a great whiskey. Try it with or without the foamy egg white top (see sidebar) and see which way you prefer!

2 tablespoons powdered allulose sweetener

1 tablespoon water

2 ounces bourbon

1 ounce fresh lemon juice

½ cup ice

1 orange slice

1 fresh cherry

1 To a small saucepan over medium heat, add powdered allulose and water. Stir until allulose is dissolved, and then remove from heat. Cool to room temperature.

2 To a rocks glass, add allulose syrup, bourbon, and lemon juice and stir to combine.

3 Add ice and garnish with orange slice and cherry. Serve immediately.

Per Serving

Calories: 141 | Fat: 0g | Protein: 1g | Sodium: 0mg | Fiber: 0g | Carbohydrates: 21g | Net Carbohydrates: 3g | Sugar: 2g

To Make This with a Foamy Egg White Top

Add the cooled allulose syrup, bourbon, lemon juice, and ½ ounce egg white to a shaker glass and shake vigorously for 30 seconds. Add the ice and shake for another 30 seconds. Strain the drink into a coupe glass and serve immediately.

Standard US/Metric Measurement Conversions

VOLUME CONVERSIONS	
US Volume Measure	**Metric Equivalent**
⅛ teaspoon	0.5 milliliter
¼ teaspoon	1 milliliter
½ teaspoon	2 milliliters
1 teaspoon	5 milliliters
½ tablespoon	7 milliliters
1 tablespoon (3 teaspoons)	15 milliliters
2 tablespoons (1 fluid ounce)	30 milliliters
¼ cup (4 tablespoons)	60 milliliters
⅓ cup	90 milliliters
½ cup (4 fluid ounces)	125 milliliters
⅔ cup	160 milliliters
¾ cup (6 fluid ounces)	180 milliliters
1 cup (16 tablespoons)	250 milliliters
1 pint (2 cups)	500 milliliters
1 quart (4 cups)	1 liter (about)

OVEN TEMPERATURE CONVERSIONS	
Degrees Fahrenheit	**Degrees Celsius**
200 degrees F	95 degrees C
250 degrees F	120 degrees C
275 degrees F	135 degrees C
300 degrees F	150 degrees C
325 degrees F	160 degrees C
350 degrees F	180 degrees C
375 degrees F	190 degrees C
400 degrees F	205 degrees C
425 degrees F	220 degrees C
450 degrees F	230 degrees C

WEIGHT CONVERSIONS	
US Weight Measure	**Metric Equivalent**
½ ounce	15 grams
1 ounce	30 grams
2 ounces	60 grams
3 ounces	85 grams
¼ pound (4 ounces)	115 grams
½ pound (8 ounces)	225 grams
¾ pound (12 ounces)	340 grams
1 pound (16 ounces)	454 grams

BAKING PAN SIZES	
American	**Metric**
8 × 1½ inch round baking pan	20 × 4 cm cake tin
9 × 1½ inch round baking pan	23 × 3.5 cm cake tin
11 × 7 × 1½ inch baking pan	28 × 18 × 4 cm baking tin
13 × 9 × 2 inch baking pan	30 × 20 × 5 cm baking tin
2 quart rectangular baking dish	30 × 20 × 3 cm baking tin
15 × 10 × 2 inch baking pan	30 × 25 × 2 cm baking tin (Swiss roll tin)
9 inch pie plate	22 × 4 or 23 × 4 cm pie plate
7 or 8 inch springform pan	18 or 20 cm springform or loose bottom cake tin
9 × 5 × 3 inch loaf pan	23 × 13 × 7 cm or 2 lb narrow loaf or pate tin
1½ quart casserole	1.5 liter casserole
2 quart casserole	2 liter casserole

Index

Stick to your keto diet WITHOUT giving up your favorite foods!

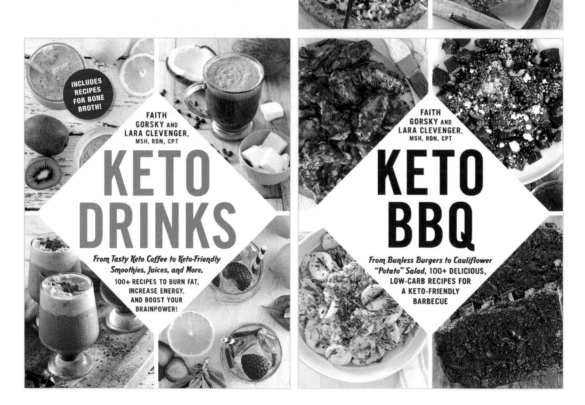

FAITH GORSKY AND LARA CLEVENGER, MSH, RDN, CPT

KETO BREAD

FROM BAGELS AND BUNS TO CRUSTS AND MUFFINS, 100 LOW-CARB, KETO-FRIENDLY BREADS FOR EVERY MEAL

INCLUDES RECIPES FOR BONE BROTH!

FAITH GORSKY AND LARA CLEVENGER, MSH, RDN, CPT

KETO DRINKS

From Tasty Keto Coffee to Keto-Friendly Smoothies, Juices, and More, 100+ RECIPES TO BURN FAT, INCREASE ENERGY, AND BOOST YOUR BRAINPOWER!

FAITH GORSKY AND LARA CLEVENGER, MSH, RDN, CPT

KETO BBQ

From Bunless Burgers to Cauliflower "Potato" Salad, 100+ DELICIOUS, LOW-CARB RECIPES FOR A KETO-FRIENDLY BARBECUE

Pick up or download your copies today!

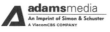